BONE

Also by the author:

Leaving My Father's House: A Journey to Conscious Femininity

The Ravaged Bridegroom: Masculinity in Women

The Pregnant Virgin: A Process of Psychological Transformation

Addiction to Perfection: The Still Unravished Bride

*The Owl Was a Baker's Daughter: Obesity, Anorexia Nervosa,
and the Repressed Feminine*

*The Maiden King (with Robert Bly): The Reunion of Masculinity
and Femininity*

*Coming Home to Myself: Reflections for Nurturing a Woman's
Body and Soul*

Now or Neverland: Peter Pan and the Myth of Eternal Youth

*Dancing in the Flames: The Dark Goddess in the Transformation
of Consciousness*

MARION WOODMAN

BONE / DYING INTO LIFE

VIKING COMPASS

A portion of the proceeds from *Bone* will be donated to the London
Regional Cancer Centre and the Canadian Cancer Society for research.

VIKING
Published by the Penguin Group
Penguin Putnam Inc., 375 Hudson Street,
New York, New York 10014, U.S.A.
Penguin Books Ltd, 27 Wrights Lane,
London W8 5TZ, England
Penguin Books Australia Ltd, Ringwood,
Victoria, Australia
Penguin Books Canada Ltd, 10 Alcorn Avenue,
Toronto, Ontario, Canada M4V 3B2
Penguin Books (N.Z.) Ltd, 182–190 Wairau Road,
Auckland 10, New Zealand

Penguin Books Ltd, Registered Offices:
Harmondsworth, Middlesex, England

First published in 2000 by Viking Penguin,
a member of Penguin Putnam Inc.

1   3   5   7   9   10   8   6   4   2

Page 246 constitutes an extension of this copyright page.

Library of Congress Cataloging-in-Publication Data

Woodman, Marion, 1928–
Bone : dying into life / Marion Woodman.
p.   cm.
ISBN 0-670-89374-9
1. Woodman, Marion, 1928—Health.   2. Cancer—Patients—Biography.   I. Title.
RC265.6.W66 A3 2000
362.1'9699471'0092—dc21
[B]   00-036787

This book is printed on acid-free paper. ∞

Printed in the United States of America
Set in Weiss
Designed by Jaye Zimet

To those who have dared the darkness,
and those who have walked with them, without pity

ACKNOWLEDGMENTS

To Ross, our family, and friends who have loved me into life
To all whose prayers accompanied me into
      the paradox of suffering—shattering into wholeness
To the medical doctors
   the alternative healers   who saved my life
     the poets and visionaries

To Michael Mendis, Susan Petersen Kennedy,
   Carole DeSanti, Tory Klose, Jaye Zimet,
      Alexandra Babanskyj and Miriam Wosk
       who patiently worked with me
To my still point that is Sophia and Christ

FOREWORD

This book is about living, not dying. It's about dying
into life. With cancer, I discovered how much dying it takes
to get here, here into my body, here onto Earth. It's about
the soul work required to heal both.

Body, like Earth, is an energy system capable not only
of nourishing itself, but also of destroying itself. With cancer, I had to differentiate the energies within myself that,
both consciously and unconsciously, led to life or death. I
have become increasingly aware of how closely connected
they are. They are no more than a heart beat apart.

For two years, I lived with cancer as an immediate part
of my daily life. I persevered in trying to experience its
many shocks as symptoms attempting to bring healing—
wholeness—into my body-soul connection. I knew I
needed the expertise of both medical science and alternative medicine to hold body and soul together. I am grateful
to both.

Since I was twelve years old, I have held body and soul
together by writing in what was once my diary, now my
journal. Confusion, grief, anger that I had learned not to
express outwardly, I discussed with myself by writing,
painting, jotting down poems and songs as they happened
inwardly. My journal became a mirror in which I could see
and hear my truth resonating in my own daily experience.

Gradually, my dreams became very important, bringing
with them dimensions I could not have imagined. They
opened another level of dialogue in which I began to experience the reality of Sophia as the Divine Mother with

whom I could build a metaphorical bridge to the Mystery that is life. My literary education, grounded in images, and my travels have made me aware that Sophia has long been a carrier of feminine wisdom by many names and for many religions.

As I grow older, issues are increasingly complex. So are my pages. New images that I don't yet comprehend, notes from friends in their own handwriting, quotations from poets articulating innuendoes of feeling, intuitive flashes— all these constitute the margins of my journal. They are like magnets that attract me to them, as a baby is attracted to a shiny or colorful object. They teach me where to find new energy for new wholeness. They are the harmonics that surround my life, hold it in a circle, waiting for the conductor to bring down the baton. Whenever that happens, it's like a divine fiat: "Be" and "It Is."

Research tells me there is no exact explanation for the "miracle of healing." It also tells me that images that feed us affect the white blood cells that strengthen the immune system. That fact, interwoven with awe at the exactness, humor, and wisdom of the inner terrain, sustains me in my solitude. Sharing my discoveries and my compassion for the sheer beauty of the human soul is my contribution to community.

If these rumblings in the margins seem disruptive to the text, then you, as reader, need not be slowed down. Skip them. The story is complete without them. You may later come back to share the expansiveness of that other dimension. But let me add a word about speed. We are now moving at a pace that is dissolving the world into an abstraction before we can take it in. If the marginalia slows you down, it is doing what I intended, knowing what it has done for me.

Practically, during my illness, one of my greatest difficulties was my inability to know what questions to ask my doctors. Fear blocked my capacity to think at my medical appointments and I would have to cobble together what I remembered of the session and what other people suggested. Just when I thought I understood where I was, another pattern of symptoms manifested, and I was once again floundering with no time to make mistakes. In *Bone*, I have included the questions that I found to be essential to my decisions. Your question may be very different, but mine may be helpful in shaping your thoughts. Once the question is in consciousness, the answer is constellated in the unconscious. Or, as I have come to understand it, the answer often lies in the unconscious waiting for the question to be consciously asked.

Bone is also about the stark truth of growing older. Sometimes in my journal, I would work very hard to figure out my responsibilities at forty, only to realize that I was now fifty, and suddenly sixty. What does it mean to be an elder in this culture? What are my new responsibilities? What has to be let go to make room for the transformations of energy that are ready to pour through the body-soul? I don't want to be here if I can't carry my own weight. As life asks new things of me, I feel I must pause, go inward, and ask, "What is my weight now? What are my new values? Who am I and not-I at this stage? Do I have the courage to live with this evolving me?"

Editing my cancer journal for publication was a very different process from the daily writing of my immediate experience. Though I was present to myself as a trained analyst as I wrote, it was not as an analyst that I was recording my experience. In editing, the analyst is more actively present, particularly in responding to the individuals' response to my depiction of them in my journal. Some of them, not surprisingly, were, at least initially, uncomfortable with their roles. Others had no difficulty relating to them. I had to reflect on the roles into which my psychic situation cast them.

I became increasingly aware in the editing that in others, "we meet ourselves in a thousand disguises." All the people, named or not named in *Bone*, are also, to some extent, inner figures who were shaping my inner life. The roles they assumed are not the lives they live independently of me. What those lives are I do not presume to know, except as they directly influence me both physically and psychically. In his memoirs, Jung confessed that other people were inalienably established in his memory "only if their names were entered in the scrolls of [his] destiny from the beginning, so that encountering them was at the same time a kind of recollection." When I first read this statement I was disturbed by Jung's seemingly inflated view of himself. Faced with the life and death issues of cancer, however, I found myself in a similar position. Those in my life who became directly involved in my now immediate situation that eclipsed all others were necessarily "entered in the scrolls of my destiny" as if they had been there from the start of my life and were there now at its possible end. "Scrolls of my destiny," hardly appropriate for most occasions, seemed accurate enough for what I now found myself in. The death advancing in my body was like a scroll as a destiny shaping my life.

In the editing, what the individuals in this journal generously offered me was their reaction to what I had written about them. In their reaction, I am better able to understand my own psychic process unfolding within what I would call a culture of cancer now consciously and unconsciously shaping the lives of millions—even those who have not been diagnosed with cancer. This psychic process remains for me a subject for analysis for the rest of my life. For better and for worse I now function within a culture of cancer whose meaning I am only beginning to understand. Certainly, it is a culture that is changing the way that all of us live. Life and death within this culture are daily being newly minted, newly understood. The myth of cancer, grounded in cancer's still far from understood physical and psychical reality, is a myth that *Bone: Dying into Life* only begins to explore. I say "myth" to include the healing fiction of the body that is its psychic truth.

The meaning of events in the moment of their happening is rarely the meaning that survives intact. In reflecting upon what I originally wrote with no thought of publication, I have been necessarily disillusioned of many of my necessary illusions. I increasingly realize that it is only through disillusionment that illusions passionately and protectively held in the moment open themselves to a reality they had blindly and defensively attempted to veil. One thing perhaps strikes me most forcibly: Cancer was once considered a sentence of death. That is how I received my own diagnosis. However hard I struggled to work positively with what medicine had to offer, something in me could not fully believe it would work. Death had taken hold of me in ways that I found difficult to fathom and even harder to overcome. At least initially, cancer presented itself to me as a way of dying rather than a way of living. Life and death were the opposites of each other, the one excluding the other. Only gradually did I realize how intimately connected they are, the one existing not in the absence but in the presence of the other. Death present in cancer was death asking to be accepted into my life.

Living with cancer as a "dying into life" still remains a way of living that I do not yet fully understand. It certainly has become an understanding of life and death that reaches beyond the medical definitions of the terms. My distrust of medicine was a trust in something more that only the presence of soul could explain. Cancer has made me sadder and wiser, and therefore richer. Because death is an essential part of life, to be fully alive is to be prepared for it. Cancer has prepared me. And that makes me grateful for my life, present to it and in it to a degree that life before cancer never attained. The gift of cancer is the gift of Now, a sense of all time precariously lodged within it. Living with death is a more abundant life.

Bone contains the marrow of my illness. In ancient Chinese paintings, rocks represent energy centers that contain the life force, *chi*, that vital energy that connects everything. Rocks, then, are the very skeleton of the Earth. *Bone* is my rock through which the Earth's vital energies flowed into new life. What I learned is the difference between destiny and fate. We are all fated to die. Destiny is recognizing the radiance of the soul that, even when faced with human impossibility, loves all of life. Fate is the death we owe to Nature. Destiny is the life we owe to soul.

BONE

November 2, 1993

Ross and I returned from England yesterday. Stayed
overnight at my studio in Toronto. Awoke in darkness,
drove home to London through November mists, watched
the dawn rise on bronze and burgundy trees.

I was not unaware that I was to meet a new doctor this
afternoon. When I checked out two tiny appearances of
blood with Dr. Cohen before we left Canada three weeks
ago, she immediately made an appointment for me with a
gynecologist for this afternoon. I couldn't do anything
about the problem right then, so it didn't spoil our trip to
Old London.

Went to Dr. Fellows at 2:00 P.M. Read *Time* magazine
until 2:25. Walked into his office. He took a sample from
my uterus, showed me little wormlike shapes bobbing in
the vial.

"Cancer," he said.

"I have terrible pain in my back," I said. "Isn't it possible
that pain could be causing the
bleeding?"

"I don't think so," he said.

"But I'm in good contact with
my body and I feel well," I said.

He left the room and returned.
"You may have misjudged this time,"
he said. "We'll send this to the lab to
be sure. . . ."

The Thought is quiet as a Flake—
A Crash without a Sound,
How Life's reverberation
Its Explanation found—

—Emily Dickinson

2:40 P.M.

Returned to the waiting room. Someone was reading *Time* magazine. I envied her innocence. "Cancer," I said to myself.

As I left the hospital, I could not connect with the thought that I had cancer. I still believed that the grinding pain of bone on bone in my back had somehow caused the bleeding. Still, I have to admit that in my imagery work I cannot make the light go through my connection to my leg on my right side. A sullen, dark weakness in the lower part of my abdomen blocks the energy.

What to do with such a blow? Drove home, told Ross. At a conscious level neither of us could take in what was happening. Will wait until next week for the verdict before beginning to worry.

November 4, 1993

Returned to Toronto, aware of not quite belonging here any longer, but still very at home in my blue, pink, mauve, and burgundy studio. Finished mail. Not worrying. In fact, the opposite is happening. That 16-year-old in me is rising up and throwing her arms to heaven and shouting, "Free at last. No one can any longer expect anything of me. I'll never have to do anything again."

My common sense tells me that's a paradoxical response to a cancer diagnosis, if indeed it is cancer. Think about that tomorrow, Scarlett Honey.

Merry weekend working at the Manhattan Center—all pink and orange and bathed in amber light. Robert Bly with his poetry and bazouki, David Whetsone with his sitar, Marcus Wise with his tabla drums, and Coleman with his poetry. What creative fun we had! Ranee's Indian dancing was profound, every finger and toe articulating the poetry as we read.

One of the poems I chose to read was "The New Rule."

It's the old rule that drunks have to argue
and get into fights.
The lover is just as bad: He falls into a hole.
But down in that hole he finds something shining,
worth more than any amount of money or power.
Last night the moon came dropping its clothes in the street.
I took it as a sign to start singing,
falling up into the bowl of sky.
The bowl breaks. Everywhere is falling everywhere.
Nothing else to do.

Here's the new rule: Break the wineglass,
and fall toward the glass blower's breath.

(Rumi, translated by Coleman Barks)

Coleman's focus was a laser beam on me. He sensed my bowl was broken. Afterward he came to me, looked straight into my eyes, held me in his arms, and never spoke.

Robert and I analyzed "The Maiden Tsar" [fairy tale] with the group. Aware of the dark feminine energy of the Baba Yaga as never before. As Death Goddess she has *fearsome* eyes.

November 7, 1993

Talked to Ross on the phone when I returned to Toronto at midnight.

"The news is not good," he said.

"Cancer?" I asked.

"Yes," he said. "I didn't want to tell you while you were in New York. The surgery will be on the eighteenth."

He had the same tone in his voice when he told me that Fraser [brother] had cancer. All the bells of Earth tolled backwards when he told me about Fraser. I don't feel that for myself. I don't feel that fatality. Thought for a long time lying in bed. Thought of how my intuitions were all operating last spring telling me to let the office go in June '93 and how I had my notification cards printed last August saying that I was closing my practice in June '94. As I designed them, I was haunted by dear Hamlet, "there's a special providence in the fall of a sparrow. If it be now, 'tis not to come; if it be not to come, it will be now; if it be not now, yet it will come: the readiness is all." I signed them "the readiness is all"!

When I went into my office last week, the violets were purple hallelujahs in the morning sun—and pink and white—but the room seemed abandoned. I think I did leave it, in spite of myself, last June.

November 8, 9, 10, 1993

I am dealing with the knowledge that I have cancer. (I have to keep telling myself that I have cancer because I feel so well, better than I have felt for two years.) After four months on crutches, I am walking again without agony in my hip and leg. I am now free to dance.

BANG! There is a loaded gun. CANCER. This time the gun is pointing at me. Hard to take that in. I deal with the knowledge by cleaning my apartment, making it as pretty as possible when I should be preparing my speech for Washington. But then, I'm not sure I am going. So I took clothes to the Goodwill, books to the secondhand shop, went to the dentist, got a new

The Soul has Bandaged moments—
When too appalled to stir—
She feels some ghastly Fright come up
And stop to look at her—

—Emily Dickinson

telephone answering machine, sent out letters to my analysands canceling sessions until Christmas, made decisions with Doris [secretary] and with Chalmers [lawyer]. Yesterday Marion [niece] came over with Aidan [grand-nephew], then came over alone today to help me get off to Washington. I am so used to doing everything for myself that it is good to have my precious niece beside me.

These are strange days, knowing I have moved into Destiny, knowing I am in exactly the right place, agonizing as it is. I think the high spirits come from that shout that rose up in me when I fell, "Free at last." I pray to God that I may live that freedom. It is very difficult to take in that one does indeed die.

As I refurbished my pinks and purples, bringing color back into my bedroom after its summer white, I did a lot of thinking. Why? Why? Why? Not why me. I feel no shame or guilt for my cancer, but that I need to take responsibility for a new future. What is the lesson to be learned here? What factors may have contributed to my dis-ease?

1. Did I betray my femininity by doing too much—too much traveling, teaching, answering mail? Was there an undercurrent whispering, "This isn't liv-

ing"? I know the weight of the mail was more than I could carry, though I love writing to my friends. Still, however much I did, always another bag turned up. The mail took two hours out of every day—two hours of making decisions, two hours that once were soul time for dancing, writing, playing.

2. Was I unable to carry the Mother projection any further? Mothering is not primary in me. I do it. I take the responsibility, the duty, the slugging density of body. I love cooking, creating beautiful space—but that is not the essential me. I do not thrive. I become a loaded-down, bloated mass. My body eventually says, "NO, I want to play." And play for me is creativity. I never played "mother" with my dolls. Moma and Topsy were my students, along with the rest of my imaginary class. In life I did not become a mother; I became a teacher. Maybe in my work I carried the Mother projection beyond the point where it was creative for me.

3. What is essential to my life is the dynamic of the archetype of Teacher/Student. When I watched Joseph Campbell come alive with light as he taught, watched his energy build instead of diminish, I knew such an archetype existed and I knew the teacher/student dynamic was my life source. My primary relationship to my father was teacher/student. The blackboard I used from four to sixteen was the focus of my constant inner dialogue, question and answer. So was the micro-

. . . if we remember the fundamental principle that the symptomatology of an illness is at the same time a natural attempt at healing. . . .

—C. G. Jung, Collected Works

scope. So now are the flip chart and colored pens. The thought of never teaching again withers me. I woke up shuddering in Zurich at the thought of never teaching creative drama again. The sheer creative delight!

4. I think my connection to that creative and spiritual source is threatened. That archetype was operative between Fraser and me; for sixty years, on and off, we were teacher/student to each other in creative relationship. As adolescents we knifed our poems on each other's doors to make sure the message was adequately received, sometimes with blood-stains for emphasis. Who knows? Who knows by what Destiny we both taught at South Secondary School in London, Ont., both directed creative drama, went our own ways, and found ourselves once again coming from different directions to the C. G. Jung Institute in Zurich and even to 223 St. Clair in Toronto after graduation. None of the moves ever seemed planned by us. But they hap-pened.

Then suddenly in '91 he had cancer. The feroc-ity of the Death Mother in destroying him, his death in '92, the shattered dream! Much as I tried—and try—to express the shock and grief, I know they linger in my body.

5. And there were other losses. Everything in me be-lieves that without consciousness there is no hope for the world. I couldn't hang on to my vision, my hope, my plan. The creativity that fed those inner fires went out, exploded into nothingness. I re-member waking up one night with a blow in the solar plexus that forced me to get up in order to breathe. My chest seemed to be pulling apart. I

tried to keep walking and dancing, but my heart was not in the movement. It was weighed down by endless contracts, the estate, taxes—so many issues that demanded energy, issues that I was no longer interested in. The immense energy that had been going out collapsed, and turned against my body.

6. I believed, and still believe, that consciousness comes both through spirit and through matter, Jung's psychoid archetype. Life has taught me that my head consciousness does not necessarily release my body consciousness. My work has taught me that I am not alone in this split. All my energy for fifteen years poured into the possibility of creating a physical space in which body could be honored equally with psyche—honored, explored, researched in terms of new scientific discoveries. However, the time was not right. God's timing and mine were not together. *Kairos* was not present.

I knew my vision of bodysoul work was not yet acceptable. I accepted that in my head. I decided to hold the tensions of the opposites until a reconciliation unknown to me found its way into consciousness in a welcoming world. I could not. However much I tried to accept this in my mind, my body, born in rejection, received it as heartbreak, which my mind interpreted as defeat. Thank God for Emily.

The physical toll was horrendous. I was simply alone. No one to talk to about the inner reality of what had happened. I needed someone who could be depended on for confi-

I fear me this—is Loneliness—
The Maker of the soul
Its Caverns and its Corridors
Illuminate—or seal—

—Emily Dickinson

dentiality. That person was Fraser. He was canny enough to see the inner dynamics, and he could keep silence.

Helga [naturopath] and Heather [body work practitioner] kept me functioning through the crisis. I remember being unable to endure the pain of hearing a lullaby—singing a baby good night. I chose to sing Fraser into the night from which he would never return.

Meanwhile my body fell into despair. Although I did all I could to release the pain, I wasn't connecting. Even my breath ceased to come in fully—as if I would break down if I really breathed, as if I would start to cry and never stop—crying for what was no longer a part of my life. "It is all right," my body said. "This is the way it is. Nothing can be done about it. I can accept it." But in accepting it, she was also withdrawing from life. In April and May she gave up any desire for food, for sexuality, for dancing. She remained very, very still. She made no effort to reach out. Even as I write that, I can feel the hand pushing down on my chest—relentless, ruthless.

November 11, 1993

John McCrae was born in Guelph, Ontario, became a physician, died in France in 1918.

At 11:00 A.M., the clocks stopped ticking as the Last Post resonated across Canada from the Ottawa cenotaph. Everyone was wearing a red poppy. Mothers, wives, daughters, lovers, weeping, forever waiting for their men to come home.

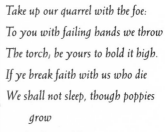

Take up our quarrel with the foe:
To you with failing hands we throw
The torch; be yours to hold it high.
If ye break faith with us who die
We shall not sleep, though poppies
grow
In Flanders Fields.

—John McCrae,
"In Flanders Fields"

November 12, 13, 14, 1993

Went to Common Boundary conference in Washington. Felt better than I have felt in years as I gave my workshop and lecture. My voice was coming from center; my full body energy was supporting it. As I stood at the podium in the soft light with all that love in front of me, I had one of those intuitive farewell flashes: "I shall never stand here again." That thought threw me into the conference with total abandon.

Conferences are being with people I love. Paula [friend] told me of the deep change that happened in her as a result of her cancer. She does not feel herself a cancer survivor. She had it cut out, and that was it. I kept telling her I do not feel sick, I do not feel I have cancer.

"Stay with that," she said. "You are not sick. You have a *health challenge.*" What a switch in thinking!

"You know, Marion," she continued, "you have for so long carried the grief and outrage of the feminine—the insult of the feminine—it's possible your body finally broke down."

Talked to Edith, who has also had cancer. She is well now. The cancer I have is encapsulated, I hope. Of course, I'm not unaware of my fear of bowel cancer. Not unaware of friends being opened up and being found full of cancer. I am not unaware of the dangers. But I hope. And I do feel well. Edith said she fought fiercely for her own time to do what she wanted to do. "Fight fiercely to defend your territory," she said.

Kathy astounded me when she read my astrology chart. "What were you doing nineteen years ago?" she asked.

"Leaving South Collegiate," I said. "In the hospital, trying to retire from teaching."

"Well, that constellation is repeating," she said. "You're maturing through your body. The mystery is working through your instrument."

"Marion," I thought, "get the message. You've got to learn to surrender to these *initiations* more cooperatively. When Sophia is moving you toward new consciousness, you need to recognize the winds of change *at once*, move with them instead of clinging to what is already gone."

Sophia is the feminine, dark, yielding, tender counterpart of the power, justice, creative dynamism of the Father.

—*Monica Furlong,*
Merton: A Biography

November 14, 1993

So I pondered all these things in my heart as I relaxed into my Victorian green coat on the front seat of the Robert Q airbus on my way home to London from Washington. Dear Ross met me, and we have been happily shopping, waiting, enjoying Windermere [condominium] and the fact that I can walk.

November 15, 1993

Need to bring the events that led up to this diagnosis into sharper focus. Need to honor the intuitive flashes from my body that I did not sufficiently receive at the time.

The first one came on ShaSha [island in Georgian Bay], where ten women were with me for an intensive in June. As we were waiting for the water taxi to take us back to the mainland, we were singing together in Miranda [cottage].

I innocently asked Jill [friend] to play "The Red River Valley." As I began to sing "From this valley they say you are going," my throat blocked, the tears came. Everyone was shocked—none more than I. I tried again, but I couldn't sing. For the first time I knew I was leaving. I knew there would never be another group there. I began to feel myself moving toward a rendezvous with Destiny, the *Titanic* and the iceberg moving inevitably toward each other. Wrong analogy! Ego submits to Fate; ego cooperates with Destiny. Consciousness makes the difference.

> Presentiment—is that long
>   Shadow—on the Lawn—
> Indicative that Suns go down—
>
> The Notice to the startled Grass
> That Darkness—is about to pass—
>
> —Emily Dickinson

Still, when I returned to London, Ross and I holidayed deliciously together at Windermere, both rather relieved to be momentarily free of worrisome motors and storm-broken trees on the island.

On July 12 Ross and I went to ShaSha together. We had two perfect days. July 14 I fell, or rather, my leg let go and I crashed on the rocks. Ross phoned the coast guard. Within half an hour the police boat splashed in; three big, handsome guys secured my leg, stretched me out into a big sling, carried me down the rocks, gently-so-gently drove the boat to Parry Sound, handed their bundle over to the waiting ambulance team, who deposited it in Emergency. Ross and I returned to the island the next day, I with my crutches.

So began the almost idyllic summer in the Lion Chair, in love with the loons, the sunrises and sunsets, and discussing with Ross his paper on the Baha'i Faith. I completely let go of everything, felt the radiance of Being. I felt no commitment to do anything, not even to entertain people who sailed in to visit. The only problem was the nights. Because I couldn't walk, fear permeated my body—a physical sensation, "Will I be able to pull the next breath in?" Came the dawn, all fear vanished.

Early September—spent a weekend in Stratford—another honeymoon—four plays in three days. Both of us were electric with poetry and became more radiant as we went from Shakespeare to Wilde and back to Shakespeare. Ross found the five perfect chairs for our dining room—antique chairs he had been looking for for thirty-five years. The grass and gardens, the direction and acting—everything perfection—except that I had to use crutches or a cane.

I have to keep coming back to my legs because I knew all was not well. Something else was moving in on me. I kept trying to boil everything down to essence. What had to go in order for me to be free was going to go. My legs were very painful, but worse, they left me vulnerable, fearful of being knocked down, unable to step out and live, to step out and dance. I felt victimized by Fate.

Victim or no victim, I went to Florida. Yes, and to California in September. (Robert and I did the opening of the *Bly/Woodman on Men and Women* films in L.A.) Had a fabulous time East and West. But, for the first time in my life, I had to sit out the whole evening of dancing. Gabrielle Roth, Dance Herself, was leading!

Then Ross and I went to London, England. Our summer had wrung out a new depth of relationship. That intensity manifested in a charged workshop on the inner marriage. We lectured together and

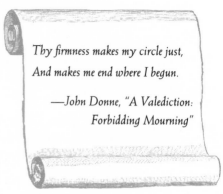

Thy firmness makes my circle just,
And makes me end where I begun.

—John Donne, "A Valediction:
Forbidding Mourning"

played together. We had three great weeks. Bruce [brother, living in England] and I had hilarious walks in Kew Gardens. The attendant graciously gave us a wheelchair; sometimes I rode and Bruce pushed; sometimes he rode and I pushed. It was excellent exercise without overexertion, but I think the Brits thought we weren't taking the wheelchair seriously enough. One intuitive moment happened when Bruce and Quint [nephew] were waving good-bye to us. Ross was pushing my wheelchair down into the tunnel that led to the plane. As I waved, I remembered Bruce saying, "When I saw Fraser going down that tunnel waving good-bye, I knew it was Good-bye."

At no time all autumn was I overworked or overlonely. I loved moving into my extraverted space; I loved seeing my analysands; I loved being alone.

The profoundest difficulty during the fall was the loss of my pearls and gold medallion watch. Part of my cleanout was my unceasing effort to find my jewels—my image of femininity, my covenant with Sophia. Repeatedly, the gut-level, bone-level emptiness when they were not where I hoped. That search continued for six weeks, until a weekend in October. I found them in the top right-hand drawer of my antique desk at Windermere. Their absence had felt like the loss of my womanhood. It prepared me for the loss of my womb and ovaries. Maybe I am losing my femininity in order to find it in another dimension.

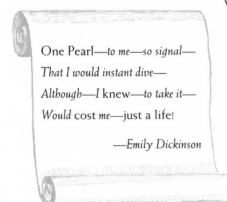

One Pearl—*to me—so signal—*
That I would instant dive—
*Although—*I knew—*to take it—*
Would cost *me—*just a life!

—*Emily Dickinson*

I have no tears, just a profound sense that this is where I am in life. Nothing can change that. It all boils down to a feeling that I have come as far as I can come on this particular path. The red light is now ON. It was, in fact, flashing last June. I always try to go that extra lap and my body goes into illness to push me out.

November 16, 1993

Tuesday—went to St. Joseph's [hospital]. Went through the preadmission program hardly knowing what I was doing. Talked to nurse, told her I thought there might be a mistake. She said to phone Dr. Fellows. Had blood and urine check and ECG. Ross came to get me as I celebrated life on the lawn with my fat bran muffin. Flowers from Bruce arrived. Yellow roses from Ross. Flowers from friends. Phone calls from all the family.

Talked to Dr. Fellows. He made it clear that I have carcinoma of the endometrium, with a three-doctor check. I made it clear to him that I am not 70—that I still have things to do with my life. All this after a yearly checkup two months ago—all clear—everything, including the Pap smear! And the green light to go ahead with hormone replacement therapy. I never quite got around to that.

November 17, 1993

Ross and I went grocery shopping today. As we drove past St. Jo's I tried to understand I was going in there tomorrow to be operated on for cancer. Dear God, it is amazing how we go about the ordinary tasks in the face of the mystery.

Did a ritual on the phone with Jean [friend] allowing my body to open to golden light.

David [nephew] came for tea and oatmeal cookies and pumpkin tarts. I am very aware how difficult this diagnosis is for the children. Cancer took both their parents. David was very quiet, his blue eyes observing everything.

The living room felt like Christmas Eve, golden with love, shimmering with a slight holding of the breath before tomorrow. Ross said, "Marion, what is going on here?" I was glad he asked the question because I too felt the extraordinary presence. So did David. I also knew there were groups and individuals praying for me right across the continent. "It must be the love that is being sent to us," I said. They agreed.

I imagined a night sky. A golden spider's web stretched endlessly, with nodules of gold connecting the filaments. I could feel the energy transmitting to London, Ont. "Dear Sophia, open me to receive it," I prayed, and felt myself totally surrender to the strength of the golden web.

Femininity is Being that knows its bone truth.

—MW

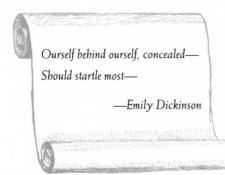

Ourself behind ourself, concealed—
Should startle most—

—Emily Dickinson

November 18, 1993
My Initiatory Dream

A ship is coming into shore bearing two pearls. I see them, I don't see them. I know they are on the ship. A 5-year-old girl, barefoot with simple dress and mop of curls, stands on deck watching. Her gaudy bracelet and corncob pipe shine in the sunlight. Behind her, a woman, young, gypsylike, barefoot, hair flowing, also watches.

These two are with me as I move into Cronedom—that queendom where I shall be free to live my own truth.

November 18, 1993

7:15 A.M.

So here on November 18, 1993, where am I? The golden sun has risen. I had no breakfast. Nothing has passed into my mouth since 8:00 P.M. last night. I am preparing my ritual. Today the doctors are going to cut out my uterus and my ovaries. This is a blood sacrifice. What does it mean? The uterus—my uterus—never bore a child. It is the physical vessel. Maybe this is the sacrifice of my feminine organs to prepare me to go the next step—to release me from all physical mothering, to release me from mothering the masses, to release me from any remaining vestige of connection to dense, opaque flesh, to release me into a new vibration in my body.

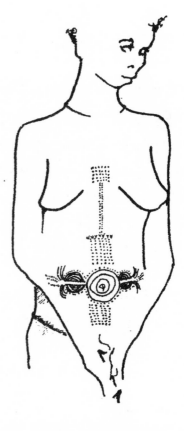

Women's scarification, "swallow" pattern. Based on a photograph in Rowe, "Abdominal Cicatrisation of the Munshi Tribe, Nigeria,"

—Bruce Lincoln,
Emerging from the Chrysalis

Cherry [sister-in-law in England] phoned yesterday. When my spirits seemed so good, she said, "Have you no grief for the loss of your womb?" "Yes," I said. (I didn't say that as I lay on the floor doing my exercises last week, I ran my fingers over my unflawed belly—"smooth as monumental alabaster"—and everything in me wept.) I am to undergo the scarification. The round belly, the navel of the world—my world—will be scarred. Yes, I do weep for the loss of my womb, my physical womb. It never had a chance to do what it would have wished to do—did wish to do: bear a child. That way my Destiny did not lie. Now it is being cut out to make room for the spiritual womb, the womb that will bear spiritual children. Lay in bed this morning blessing it before it went.

10:05 A.M.

Just completed ritual of farewell to my womb, my ovaries, to mothering the masses, to holding on to mother power. Feel a huge freedom. I pray to be opened to spiritual birthing, to the energy of my own life, to the vibration of my own new body. I pray to be totally open to the love I will receive this afternoon. I pray too that Ross will experience that love.

> Four lines cut at puberty make a woman the guardian of fertility and well-being, heir of the past and creator of the future. The scars themselves are simultaneously the means of her transformation and the visible mark that this transformation has been completed, making each girl a woman and a sacred object for all to see.
>
> —Bruce Lincoln,
> Emerging from the Chrysalis

MIDNIGHT

This afternoon Ross and I came to St. Jo's, both strong. I had one faltering moment when I picked up his little maroon case that I was taking and realized that I was going to St. Jo's to be operated on for cancer. This is the beginning of a road whose end is unknown and totally known. Ross insisted I have a private room. And so we came to 301.

I undressed and put on the floppy blue hospital gown. We talked quietly until we heard the cart rumbling in the hall. It had come for me. I got on it. Ross kissed me. He was pale as death. The orderly said he could come as far as the surgery. He came. We went down in the elevator. "You can come no further," the orderly said to Ross. The doors swung open and shut.

Dr. Sutherland introduced himself as the anesthetist. "Good Scot, " I thought. "Conscientious." Dr. Fellows introduced himself again. At 4:40 my limbs loosened, my body let go. I was gone.

A doubt if it be Us
Assists the staggering Mind
In an extremer Anguish
Until it footing find.

An Unreality is lent,
A merciful Mirage
That makes the living possible
While it suspends the lives.

     —Emily Dickinson

Sometime I came to in the intensive care unit. Ross was there. Then sometime I opened my eyes in 301, exhausted but OK. The nurse gave me a button to push when I needed painkiller. Bouquet arrived from Bruce—it brings life to the brown wood of the room. Two pink ginger blossoms, one leaning down to greet the other—Japanese style on a red tray—with the "earth" full of small, dark purple orchids, shiny foliage, and three lilies ready to burst.

November 19, 1993

Woke up this morning with the realization that my belly has been scarified. It hurts when I walk in the corridor, rolling the IV pump beside me.

Flowers from Sylvia and Pam. One red rose from Susan.

Rosa, my nurse, is beautiful—plump, exquisite eyes, innocent, strong—as I once

scared—
  scarred—
    sacred—

was. I could not see my own beauty when I was her age, but I certainly see hers.

Another nurse woke me up in the night to show me how to work the painkiller contraption.

"I know how to use it," I said.

"Then why don't you use it?" she snapped.

"I don't need it," I replied. "I'm using imagery."

"Oh?" was her only response. I knew she had written me off as a New Age flake.

November 20, 1993

More flowers today. No desire to move much. Feeling more pain and sheer weakness as I try to keep walking. The carts keep coming and going past my door.

In love with my flowers and the dear ones who sent them. Throughout these three days at St. Jo's I have clung to these flowers whenever I have felt I am nobody. They are the love; they are the beauty in life. Many times I have wakened in the night and breathed them in as I listened to the hospital sounds—the stifled sobs in the corridors, the gentle cadences of nurses' voices.

Sunday. Opening out to life again.

Jill sent me a little white buffalo with turquoise eyes. I hold it in my hand to feel the Navaho energy pouring through me from the earth into the sky and back into my heart. My friends are incredible. To feel myself the cup into which all this earthly love flows, the cup through which it flows and rises to the brim and overflows into Sophia's laughter, filling the universe with rain and rivers and flowers—and my heart with vibrant peace.

"Yea, though I walk through the valley of the shadow of death. . . ." Dear Sophia, how the cycle spirals and swings into wider spirals and how your love holds the spiral true in my heart.

Mary [friend] arrived with yellow lilies this morning. My whole body leapt up to greet her. So glad to be alive to meet her. She thinks I've taken in too much poison. Now the sacrifice for the feminine has been made and we will get on with our work. Her card of the dancers in space is so right. The placement of the energy in their

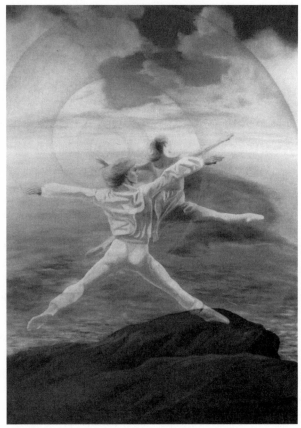

From "Infinite Journey," oil painting by Gloria Joy.

bodies is exact—embodied dancers, not disembodied angels.

Elinor [friend] arrived just after Mary left. She bore a great garbage bag with something heavy—a hibiscus plant—three of them, from Marcella [friend]—Mother, Virgin, Crone. She also brought a bag of Body Shop ointments and powders to soothe my soul. Softness enveloped the room. She talked about my not mothering anymore, about accepting my freedom to live my own life. We walked in the corridor, free now of the IV pump.

Ross came. Read Baha'i prayers together. "Together" is the crucial word. Feel so cared for and protected in the hospital.

> Thy name is my healing, O my God, and remembrance of Thee is my remedy. Nearness to Thee is my hope, and love for Thee is my companion. Thy mercy to me is my healing and my succor in both this world and the world to come. Thou, verily art the All-Bountiful, the All-Knowing, the All-Wise.
>
> —Baha'u'llah, *Prayers and Meditations*, CLXX

November 22, 1993

Cleaned my flowers, blessed them in their going or coming, packed Ross's little maroon case, was ready when he came at noon. Drove home through the sparkling wintry morning.

The house is golden. Ross and I are happy to be

here together. Karen sent royal golden pears from Oregon—Harry and David's. Ross and I had one for lunch between us—dessert for eight days. Simplicity. Helps me to focus.

Starting to work on what to do now. The surgery is over. The death is complete. Out of death comes new life. But I have no idea what to do to help myself, what to eat, how to exercise. Have begun to realize that I have cancer and will probably have to work at this for the rest of my life. Elizabeth phoned to ask if I would talk to a medical doctor interested in alternative methods. "Yes," I said. Others phoned. Beginning to feel deluged with possibilities of what to do—clinics in the States and Mexico, New York specialists, macrobiotic diets, colonics, healers. I don't know.

Put flowers in every room. Take delight every morning in giving them fresh water, cutting their stems, seeing their faces—especially now the lilies with their sexy stamens and pistils—the whole of the life process involved. In their gradual opening, singing their glorias, they are magnifying God. And then the inevitable transparency in their petals as they change color, and the greater transparency requiring a different container to mirror the dignity of their fading. Then their silent letting go. I need to treasure them through their entire cycle of birth, blossoming, full radiance, and gradual return to death. I can thank them, bless them, and let them go. The hour I spend with them every morning is healing for me. Zen and the Art of Flower Arranging.

> *A sepal, petal, and a thorn*
> *Upon a common summer's morn—*
> *A flask of Dew—a Bee or two—*
> *A Breeze—a caper in the trees—*
> *And I'm a Rose!*
>
> —*Emily Dickinson*

November 24, 1993

Without the love, would I bother? Without Ross, would I care? More and more, I feel the initiation—the letting go of something that is finished in order to move into new life. How to let go? How to be sure at the unconscious level that I am letting go? Consciously, I let go the instant I fell last July, but as I sat in the Lion Chair the letting go was the letting go of life itself, rather than the letting go of the part that had become destructive. The bliss masked the despair. Unconsciously I was confusing the actual and the metaphorical. I know I am dealing with the Great Mother in her death aspect. In the past she could hypnotize me, blind me to my unconscious death wish in bingeing and starving. Now again. I have to turn her face around and feel myself looking into the eyes of the loving Mother. How to be sure I am moving from the negative face of the arche-type to the positive? That has to happen, but it is hard to recognize the move when the dark face is so locked, so fierce, and so fiercely locked in the unconscious.

I have carried this dark load too long. I am delivered of a very dark, dead baby. If I cannot get hold of the positive side of the archetypal dimension of this, I think I will die. And that dimension has to do with the emergence of the Virgin bride at a new height and new depth on the spiral. Very aware now that the spiral—the movement of the Virgin Gypsy of my initiatory dream—is a double helix. As above, so below.

Please, God, let me live the Spiritual Warrior, fighting for the new order. Dear Sophia, let your

Thou who art terrible,
Thou who art eternal . . .
Thou who art the moon and the
   moon's light
And happiness itself . . .

—Ajit Mookerjee,
Kali: The Feminine Force

radiance release me into Virgin/Crone. Masculine and feminine together, we may make the transition.

November 25, 1993

Ross was very reluctant to take me to see Helga [naturopath] and Zeca [naturopath]. From his point of view this is medical time 100 percent. He was quiet, withdrawn as we drove to Toronto, and held back as I got out of the car to go into the office. I was so glad to see Helga. My body leapt into her arms and I assured her I was not going to die and she reassured me. We talked mostly about the operation and future procedures. She gave me essiac, Nurse Caisse's cancer remedy, as several of my friends had so vehemently suggested. She also gave me remedies for detoxifying the liver and gallbladder, and building the immune system.

I felt strong when I went into Zeca's office. He listened to my story and showed no fear, but said we'd get on with the healing. We talked about my connection to Fraser, my loss of purpose, my being constantly in the collective. All of these factors he considered, then gave me a powerful treatment. He checked out my body responses, gave me remedies.

I listened to the chanting on the sound system and lay there accepting the healing. I stepped out into Yorkville ex-

Homeopathy never deals with an overt disease manifestation—with an infection, shall we say—but with that disturbance which enables the infection to take hold, *contains* it, as it were, as a partial element. It does not deal with an effect of changed chemistry, but with that energy, that ordering element, which permits this change of chemistry to occur.

—*Edward C. Whitmont,*
Psyche and Substance

panding into Christmas. All the lights were burning white in the trees; it seemed a Heaven on Earth. I seemed to float above the lights, vibrant, scintillating. Ross picked me up. I told him all that had happened. He was quite silent.

Then Martin [medical doctor, close friend for fifty years] came over on Saturday night and Ross told him about Zeca. Martin was furious, as I knew he would be. This guy in Toronto—he'd like to have his name and he would report him—a charlatan. He paced around the living room working himself into a real frenzy of contempt, at the same time satisfying Ross as he got hotter and hotter. I sat quietly in the chair realizing that all the time I have been talking about cherishing my femininity, loving Sophia, honoring Her, he must have thought it was words, words, words. How differently we think in spite of forty-five years of dialogue! In the crunch nothing existed in his mind but medical science, and my more feminine world was hocus-pocus. He was certain Martin would clarify and I would abjure "this rough magic" (*The Tempest*). The wilder Martin got, the quieter I became. I knew there was no sense trying to persuade him. I knew he was trying to protect me; I felt I would die for sure if I betrayed Sophia. After Martin left, I simply told Ross I was going to continue going to Toronto once a week on the bus.

"You can't do that!" he said. "Now we're going from London to Toronto every week, instead of you coming from Toronto to London. When is this 401 [highway between London and Toronto] going to stop? The corridor in our new apartment will replace the 401, but when?"

"I don't care," I said. "I will continue to go where my soul is recognized."

"I understand that, Marion," he said, "but you can't split like this."

"I'm not a bit split," I said. "Medical science can do its best for me and naturopathy can do its best. I'll take the best of both worlds."

So I work with diet and detox and remedies to build my immune system. Very helpful books from Larry Dossey, Jeanne Achterberg, Bernie Siegel. I am honored that they consider me a friend. I put my own hot hands on my belly and bring in light and heat. I'm no good at *fighting* cancer cells. I can't use a gun or wild dogs or spitfires. Those images do not work for me. But I can suffuse darkness with light, and I do, three or four times a day, and often in the night.

> . . . the unconscious and automatic functions become related to an ego center and thus attain an entirely new quality, consciousness.
>
> —*Edward C. Whitmont,*
> Psyche and Substance

November 28, 1993

Ross's birthday. William Blake's birthday. Two rebel souls barely on this earth! Last year Ross's 70th. So glad we celebrated with our friends, because I couldn't have done anything this year. But last year Marion and I had such fun cooking and baking for all the guests. I made five Viennese Sacher tortes—the birthday cake I've made for Ross every year of our married life. Seventy white roses and seventy white candles! Windermere glowed with poetry, music, and dance.

Well, that was last year. This year three white candles in three glass candlesticks. No Sacher torte; no less love. Robert and Marguerite [friends] delivered a delicious birthday dinner and graciously left us alone. We talked of other birthdays—an almost inevitable sense of summing up. I was aware of our journey together. Both of us have a certain sense of detachment—a looking at the Divine Comedy and seeing each other as the soul God gave us with whom to share the journey. Quite apart from the fact that Ross is my husband, I see the dignity of his soul—proud, receptive, compassionate—always making place for beauty, music, art—expressions of soul in himself and others. I am equally aware of his 71 years, his frailty, his recently diagnosed diabetes. He is "cleared" by the prayers of my friends as I am. As I lay receiving the energies the other night, I felt the shimmer in my body and the letting go—the clearing. When I came back into the living room, he too had felt the clearing.

November 29, 1993

Went yet again to see our possibly new condominium on Sydenham Street. Time really closing in, and I cannot help feeling that place is mixed up in our future for better or for worse, and it could be for worse. I do have cancer. I may never be able to move. Doesn't matter. Ross has been looking at it repeatedly for three years. Sydenham is in his heart, and I will never forget how my heart soared when the real estate woman said, "Now or never, Ross." I felt the release from Highway 401, from the train and the bus. I felt Destiny once again pounding on the door. Decision now. Yes, you are just home from the hospital. Yes, the new home is there. Yes, there is room for your office. Move into the new life. That is where it is to happen. High ceilings, light, a garden, fresh air, fresh sunlight, new hope.

November 30, 1993

Signing Day. Sydenham is ours.

Staying with how purposeful I feel. I still have work to do. I have to be careful reading cancer material because I don't feel I am moving toward death. I feel no pain or weakness. I am reconstructing my life and getting on to new work. I am looking ahead. That's why I could so quickly say, "Yes, let's take Sydenham."

Joy in today. *Re-member* myself. Paula said everyone at the imagery conference stressed the importance, in those who survived, of their sense of purpose. That's what I had lost—my sense of purpose. I was dis-membered, lost center. Now I am re-membering, gathering together the prodigal parts of myself and welcoming them home.

> This body is no longer as usual: it is scarcely more than a center of concentration . . . it is not a skin-bound body. . . . It's a sort of aggregate, a concentration of vibrations.
>
> *—Mother, quoted in Satprem,* The Mind of the Cells

December 1, 1993

A new month. My God, what did go on in November? Talked to Marion. She and Kathryn [niece-in-law] have decided that Christmas will be at Marion's this year—and no big Christmas breakfast. Just the afternoon and dinner.

We will all give soul gifts to each other—a poem, a song, a dance. No one has any extra money, so this is the way to have a loving Christmas with no financial suffering afterward.

I began the move this morning. Cleaned cupboards. Anything dispensable went either into the garbage or into a pile for Goodwill or into a small pile to be considered later.

Got caught in old photographs, worked on them most of the day and into the night. Sheer delight! Kept all the ancient sepia pictures—weddings, children, ancestral families. Ross came and went. Looked at hundreds of slides—relived our trips, unique moments in our lives, of interest only to us. Kept the ones that are good photographs. Made carousels for each of the children from their infancy to now, family picnics, Christmases, birthdays. "One generation passeth away, and *another* cometh. . . . The sun also ariseth" (Ecclesiastes 1:2–5).

The accident of cleaning out a
drawer
Brings the tragedy home,
though with it
The vast redemptive process
of small, familiar things.

—Ross Woodman

Sat by the fireplace, re-membered each picture, from my parents' courting days right through to now, sacrificed most of them to the fire. No place to store seven big boxes of albums that no one will ever look at again. Needed my golden sword with a silver handle—masculine gold with feminine silver—sharp discrimination with infinite love. Only essentials are going to the new house.

Some grief in disposing of the old albums, but feel I have brought my life line into sharper consciousness within myself. For the first time I saw the inherent energy in my adolescent face. Bubbles, my friends called me. The wild long curly hair that is so fashionable now! The flawless skin!

I was so trapped in my "fatness" I saw none of that. The solid line throughout was my trying to make space to fly and forever smashing my wings against the bars of the cage. Granted, the cage grew bigger and very big, but I was always beyond the collective in my soul and always cut back by the collective in my body.

December 2, 1993

   More work with the albums. Also began writing Christmas cards. "Seamless" is the picture this year, chosen in September from our summer photos. Marion wasn't sure she liked its shadows at all, nor did she like the photo of my empty rocking chair with my straw hat. Several of my summer photos had a presentiment of death in them. Of course, being on crutches did not enhance my sense of leaping into life. But I knew something was gone, forever gone—and that knowing came out in my pictures and songs. It also came out in my sense of birthing into Stratford. Such a leap into Shakespeare I have never felt before—and that is a momentous statement. This time I could not get enough.

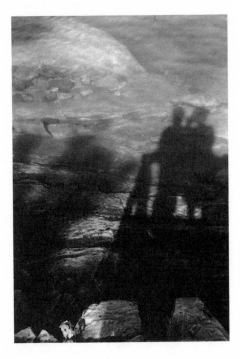

   To some friends we wrote, "We chose this card in September. We called it 'Seamless' because we could not see where the water connected to the land, nor whither the great depths led. Now, *Seamless*

of course, 'seamless' resonates with deeper resonances, resonances that have to do with temporal meeting eternal, substance meeting shadow."

To other friends, who knew us as Nagg and Nell in the garbage cans in Beckett's *Endgame*, we wrote:

> Nell to Nagg: It was deep, deep. And you could see down to the bottom. So white. So clean.

That too has the eternal ring at the center of the temporal. *Essence*. It astonishes me over and over again how my body and psyche knew that a death was taking place but my ego could not accept the message. My leg was telling me in no uncertain terms that I could not go on at the office. But I kept trying. Instead of getting better, it got worse after the initial healing. Then it genuinely improved in England. Its purpose was complete. It did get me to Dr. Cohen, and thence to Dr. Fellows. When the cancer was detected, my leg no longer was in pain.

December 3, 1993

. . . Only I discern—
Infinite passion, and the pain
Of finite hearts that yearn.

—Robert Browning,
"Two in the Campagna"

Taking daily walks in the halls. Too cold and icy to go outside. Don't want to fall and break my surgery open. Somehow, Ross and I don't seem able to get our tree up for Christmas. We talk about it. I look at the baubles, but there is something in both of us that is not challenging Fate. We're not letting ourselves hear inner voices: "This might be our last tree, our last Christmas together." So we say,

"We'll be in Toronto for Christmas," and light the candles on the mantelpiece.

Susan arrived with a bright red pot of soup, and Dianne with bowls of tasty green and yellow veggies. Mary strode into the kitchen bearing aloft "a happy chicken from the organic co-op, one who never knew a wire cage." So thankful not to have to cook.

December 6, 1993

Dr. Fellows phoned this morning. Bad news. The operation was not as successful as he had hoped. Report from the lab shows the cancer had perforated the uterine wall. No lymph nodes were taken out to check, so we don't know if the lymphatic system is clear or not. He suggested I go to the clinic for further treatment.

Hung up the phone. Stared at my azalea. Prayed to Christ to help me put on the full armor of God. A new wind blows. I need my Spiritual Warrior, free of any allegiance to the Old King.

December 10, 1993

Ross and I went to the clinic—as attractive and light as a big C waiting room could be. We went in together to meet the specialist—young, piercing blue eyes, suave. He had my report in his hand.

"What's this Chungian analyst?" he asked.

"Five years' training in Zurich at the C. G. Jung Institute," I said. "Jung was a student of Freud until they quarreled."

"Oh, yes," he said. "Dreams and all that kind of thing."

I felt his dismissal; I made no response.

He took a brief history of the cancer and said we'd be setting up some radiation—five weeks, five times a week and a forty-eight-hour session in the hospital at the end.

"We'll think about that session at the end," I thought. "I have a naturopath," I said.

"Aren't you lucky!" he said, somewhere between a snicker and a snarl.

"Yes," I said, "I am." He knew I meant it. "Can you tell me how to prepare for this radiation?" I asked. "Nutrition?"

"Know nothing about it," he said. "That's not my field."

We left. Drove home in silence. Went to bed.

December 11, 1993

One-hour phone conversation with Jean. Together we entered a "new universe"—the cosmos as a flower, God as the gardener. She explains archetypes as energy templates, seeds that are coded with potential energies, sacred geometry. Planting a seed, actual and metaphorical, is sacred work because the mystery of the code is beyond us. The field of space and time is invisible, but in that space and time is the conscious awareness of the mind of the universe. Within it are mystical experience and high loving. The cosmos, the flower, is being created in its entirety every ecosecond. We are working with God in a process of coevolution.

In our generative ground of matter, we human beings are moving into a recognition of the whole kingdom of heaven. That recognition is demanding major leaps

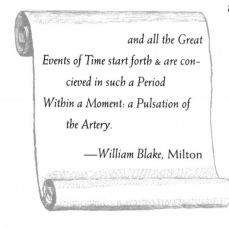

and all the Great Events of Time start forth & are concieved in such a Period Within a Moment: a Pulsation of the Artery.

—William Blake, Milton

out of the old forms of the paradigms, especially out of archaic patriarchal forms, old physical forms, and outworn perceptions. We are still identified with the original seed, but something more refined, more subtle is emerging. "High tech and high soul," says Jean, "a global mind field that enhances the world—pollination, cross-fertilization, acceptance of new images." Old membranes will break down in order to allow the new to come in; hence, so many illnesses as the old immune system writhes under the stress of the new physical, mental, spiritual pressures.

The goal in this immense shift is the integration of consciousness and matter, each supporting the other in its ascent toward unity. Insight, empathy, meaning are in this mutual ascent. The deep metaverse is unified awareness; differentiation supports that unification. In the move toward unity, we will move through continuous birth, death, rebirth patterns. All is energy in motion. All flowers compose one garden. All are part of this mutual ascent.

In this reconstruction of mind/body, radical freedom of choice is ours—freedom to make our mistakes, freedom to suffer because we try to force what is too big into what is too small. To move into the new, we will allow Being, Body, Mind to flow through us. Holographic change is an immense cosmic law.

Ablaze, I put down the phone. Jean, Jean, thank you for helping me to re-member myself. My work is more connected to shadow than yours, but now I re-member my vision. You reconnected me to one of my templates. Images are pouring through me. I see workshop after workshop in Toronto in which Michele or Bev or David and I are working with groups on dreams in relation to body work week after week, year after year, consciousness and matter each supporting the other in mutual ascent and descent toward unity.

I see analysands with different illnesses caused by the breakdown of their immune systems, at the same time struggling in their dreams to break out of the patriarchal prisons that disempowered them, struggling to take the wire clamps off their mouths. I see them too through long hours of painful differentiation and immense patience, holding the tension of seeming opposites until a new third reveals an inner unity.

Yes, and I see the intensives with Mary, Ann, and Paula, the participants—some pounding their fists on the floor in rage, others sobbing out the heartbreak of a lifetime—going through death and reentering life at a new level of consciousness. Every ecosecond is new. We are working with Sophia in a process of coevolution.

And I think of the workshops with Robert where the tension between the men and women becomes so intense that we think it best to separate so that individuals within their own gender groups may find their own energy codes. Then they can express them through body in order to bring them to consciousness and, in that process, bring them to a more subtle civilized level. That subtlety comes out in the poetry, music, dancing, the "high loving" of a group that has worked through its differentiation to a place of unity.

Jean, again thanks for rekindling my spirit, my vision. I know this is my path. I know this death I am going through has to do with matter that cannot move as quickly as the consciousness that inhabits it. Too much light in too dense matter. My dreams have been telling me

"Jung's method, which bestows universal validity on archetypes and the collective unconscious, is linked to the idea of imagination as participation in the truth of the world."

—Italo Calvino,
Six Memos for the Next Millenium

that for a year. I am in radical process. The culture is in radical process. Maybe I, like so many others, am a microcosm of the macrocosm. Maybe my exhaustion mirrors the exhaustion in the soul of the culture. Maybe I need to lie fallow, rest, and allow the new growth to happen. No goals, no agendas. Be open-ended in order to allow anything to come in through experience, through dreams, through a totally new sense of reality. As Jean puts it, "The Australian Aborigines have 'low tech, high soul.'"

That reminds me of Anthony's [psychiatrist's] story about his beloved Australia, that story we were going to tell in the book we never wrote about healing from two perspectives—the allopathic and the soul-centered. It is a true story, but I may not have all the details exact.

Anyway, an Australian documentary team challenged the Aborigines to take on a top unit in the Australian army in a race to see who could reach a remote spot in Queensland first. Both accepted the challenge. Both teams arrived at the starting point. The army was laden down with heavy trucks full of cartons of food, compasses, instruments necessary to cut through woods, walkie-talkies, and every possible high-tech device. The Aborigines arrived laughing and dancing, each wearing one piece of clothing and carrying one long spear. Intrigued by the army's gear, they also teased them about their maps. "Not that way," they said. "Sacred forest. You can't go through there."

"Sacred forest, indeed!" The army officers laughed.

So they set out. The army, having figured out the shortest, swiftest way, launched out toward the sacred forest. The natives laughed and danced behind them. Sure enough, the profane army trucks drove into sacred mud, sacred quicksand, and had to be laboriously towed out as the lithe little bodies danced and laughed, making no effort to get on with their own journey. They pointed the army driv-

ers in the right direction and then headed off on an opposite route.

Television cameras accompanied both; two camps were
pitched each night. The soldiers, exhausted from their journey, got out their cartons and tin cans, and listlessly ate.
The natives waited until sunset, then danced their way out
to sea on a fallen tree, extended their exquisite bodies,
black against the orange sky, and, creating a perfect line,
raised their spears, caught their fish, took them to shore to
cook and eat. And then to sleep. Perhaps they arrived
in Queensland, perhaps not. No matter. "Low tech, high
soul."

December 12, 1993

The *ifs* in the radiation conflict are strong. I dialogue
with the two sides, but always come back to "*If* I had
enough courage, *if* I had total
trust, *if* I had invincible faith, I
wouldn't subject my body to this
torture."

Talked to Jean again. She
thinks the *if* is a bridge word, attempting to join the three parts
of my brain. Right now my rational brain is doing all the work.
Be careful, Marion. There are two
other more primitive brains that
are trying to be heard. They have
a wisdom of their own. Meditation is one way to reach
them. Trance is another. Jean is going to help me make the
bridge on Saturday. She and Ellen offered to come here on
Valentine's Day for a healing session.

I look forward to knowing how you
deal with your responsibilities. But
you won't anticipate an answer: the
answer will present itself, provided
you don't insist upon certainty.

—*Dr. E. A. Bennet, Letter,* 1972

Says Jean, "The new mythology is sizzling. *Breakdown* in order to *break through*." She affirms so many of my so-called far-out ideas about femininity. Nothing far-out about them! They are deep within and they are manifesting whether the collective accepts them or not. The Black Madonna is pushing through from the unconscious in dreams. She is bringing the living feminine into everyday planetary life; no longer can she be frozen into a goddess on a pedestal or a goddess in bed. She utterly rejects patriarchal projections that chain her in stereotypes—naïve victim, stupid, melodramatic, histrionic, hysterical—all those words that have imprisoned her, reduced her to silence. She will no longer be silent. There is no turning back. She strides into dreams rich and juicy, full of fun and vibrant sexuality and intense spirituality—all One.

Within themselves, men are recognizing her fine tuning in feeling and sensibility. They know she must be honored in equal partnership with masculinity. The polarities that create hostility between men and women are archaic, like so many other polarities.

In seeing beyond those polarities, we cherish the diversity of the whole of creation. We celebrate the One who contains them all. Talk about the global village is still talk. Until we are able to perceive through feminine eyes, to embody our femininity, we cannot hold the opposites without opposition. We cannot live the Oneness of the feminine.

Jean thinks I have taken on "the incarnation of possibility." For sure, I have blown out the old human circuits. Through my experiences in India, through my illnesses and dreams, I have left behind the world I was born into. I resonate with a new vision in my cells, see with different eyes, and hear with different ears. So long as I trusted my own relationship to the Divine Feminine by keeping silent and living her reality inwardly, I could move with fluidity in both the inner and outer worlds. I can remember feeling the metabolism in my cells go up, being pushed to let past perceptions go, recognize new ones, and realize them in my body. Once I began to voice this inner reality, the interface between me and outer reality became more difficult.

My spiritual womb is now my place of gestation. As a human being I am gestating possibility, trying to connect to the new images arising from the archetypal field, and trying to incarnate their energy into my daily life. I am trying to be as faithful as possible to my own evolving process. Sometimes my process is radically out of balance—my spiritual knowing is far beyond my body's capacity to incarnate it. Body is much slower to give up the past—old fears of not pleasing others, old eating patterns, old patterns of relationship. I have a Jaguar engine in a Volkswagen chassis. I know the power of the engine could destroy the chassis. The images that come from my spiritual womb hold the energy that can destroy or heal. They hold the transformative power that connects body, soul, and spirit. Internalizing the images, breathing, dancing, writing them into my body, giving them time to radiate my cells with new energy—that is healing. I know this is true, but I have to keep saying it to myself. Too often my crocodile says, "Just go to sleep, Marion. Forget it!"

December 13, 1993

Dearly Beloved, to the radiance of your beauty, I surrender. May my Being be complemented in your resonance. Is Death but another frequency?

Some of my roses are no longer able to hold up their heads, so I cut them off and put them individually in champagne glasses with fern. Others are taking on the silver sheen of age, so I put them in pewter. Their love and the love of those who sent them radiate through every room and through my body. I look at the beauty of the blossoms and let them *be* as they move into transparency and die. Death is part of life.

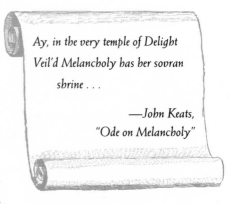

Ay, in the very temple of Delight Veil'd Melancholy has her sovran shrine . . .

—*John Keats,* "Ode on Melancholy"

Naomi and Marlene sent us a video of Fonteyn and Nureyev dancing *Romeo and Juliet.* Fantastic! Each fully resonating the other! I remember Fonteyn in 1953, when she was supposedly ending her brilliant career. She was exquisite, a technically perfect doll, sparkling like a diamond. Then, oh could we ever forget that night at Covent Garden in 1962, the first appearance of Fonteyn with the Tartar who had defected from Russia. Fonteyn was younger than I had ever seen her, all woman, all vitality, her body so alive it radiated light. Nureyev's leopard energy transfixed the audience.

When I dance with Fonteyn, it is different. There is one aim, one vision. There is no tearing us apart.

—*Nureyev,* The New York Times, *1970*

Together they were one body with two energies. Sheer magic! The curtain calls were an orgy of clapping and crying, waterfalls of daffodils pouring over the balconies from the jardinieres in the foyer. And all the evenings of dance that followed. How lucky we were to be in London that year! How incredible our journey has been—"for better, for worse . . . in sickness and in health . . . till death us do part."

December 14, 1993

Christmas is approaching. No parties this year, no shopping, no pressure. Time to contemplate the coming of the new consciousness: "How silently, how silently/The wondrous gift is given."

Turn on the TV and a totally other reality crashes in—Barbie dolls, Barbie with a boyfriend, fifty possible menus for the festive season, and how many possible outfits? Our culture is schizophrenic, broken into autonomous parts. Is cancer a *reaction* to that splitting all around us? Is it an attempt to find oneness another way? Is it also a *response* to that splitting—concretized poison in a tumor?

So fair a fancy few would weave
In these years! Yet, I feel,
If someone said on Christmas Eve,
"Come, see the oxen kneel,

"In the lonely barton by yonder coomb
Our childhood used to know."
I should go with him in the gloom,
Hoping it might be so.

—Thomas Hardy, "The Oxen"

December 16, 1993

Living for this moment. NOW. Not the past, not the future. Singing the Hallelujah Chorus—NOW. Feeling my Beloved Spirit dancing with my Soul, singing the words, transporting us to laughter and dance. Transporting, yes—

leaving behind compression, depression, repression. Dancing into EXPRESSION. How my body sings!

Let it out. Be FREE. Be Bubbles again. I am Bubbles so long as I am in my body, feeling my 16-year-old strength and Leo mane of curly hair. Movement and laughter are my delight. Bubbles is reemerging in my dreams, pitching aside the clutter in my life, knowing her own voice and her own time for her own needs. "Here I am," she says. Bubbles could teach Barbie a lot about singin' the Blues.

December 18, 1993

Returning to my self-discipline routine. Taking time and energy to do my exercises, walking half an hour every day, and gently dancing. Not relying on housework to give me the exercise I need. Feeding myself the vitamins and remedies Zeca gave me, green and yellow steamed vegetables, drinking eight glasses of pure water. Not begrudging myself the rest I need. Visualization and meditation holding the days and nights together.

Feeling new self-respect for my body. Realize I had lost my freedom in it. It had become a heavy load to carry. Part of this heaviness was too much responsibility, too much absorption in details, too many burdens that were not mine. I remember myself in London, England, when we were on sabbatical—free, free as light and air, free to adventure and live life's surprises. Part of that lightness is as simple as getting enough fresh air. Without oxygen my metabolism slows down. I retain water. I

Mysticism must rest on crystal clear honesty, can only come after things have been stripped down to their naked reality.

—*Etty Hillesum*, An Interrupted Life

carry my own unshed tears in my thighs, and the tears of others. Remember Frankl's story, Marion. When he was in the concentration camp, he was the only one who could still put on his boots. When the others with their swollen feet asked him how that was possible, he said, "I cry all night."

This walk with Death makes me realize yet deeper that there is no freedom without discipline—physically, emotionally, spiritually.

Dear Sophia, let me be your disciple. Let me be your pupil. Let me look into your pupils and see myself reflected there. Let me be disciplined in your love. The more I accept your discipline, the deeper is my love for you.

December 19, 1993

Dreamed of running into the arms of my Beloved—a dream as erotic as it was spiritual. Total surrender!

Am very aware of the "Jingle Bells" of Christmas that no longer ring for the new life that brings the new consciousness— the Baby born of a surrendered Virgin. How else but through them can we dare to keep living in a crumbling culture? The Virgin walks one step at a time without knowing the goal. She can stay in life, even see the beauty in life in spite of the crumbling, because she can open to spirit. Cancer is taking you to a level of surrender you never imagined, Marion. In your crumbling, be

When Merton asked a Buddhist abbot, "What is the knowledge of freedom?" the abbot replied, "One must ascend all the steps, but then when there are no more steps one must make the leap. Knowledge of freedom is the knowledge, the experience, of this leap."

—*Marion Woodman,*
The Pregnant Virgin

conscious of the Virgin's voice, "Be it unto me according to thy word" (Luke 1:38).

December 20, 1993

Ross and I came to my studio in Toronto this morning. Instantly strung the balcony lights, set the figures of our forever crèche in evergreen with white candles, fixed the flowers I had brought from home, and relaxed into our thirty-fifth wedding anniversary. Ross lying on the couch reading, the choir from King's College Chapel, friends phoning, finishing the Christmas cards. Thankful there are no exams to mark as there always used to be on this special night. Ross will broil our anniversary fillets wrapped in bacon. My wedding gown isn't here, so I'm not anxious wondering if I'll be able to zip it up this year.

The marriage we have is not the marriage we committed to thirty-five years ago. Sure, the storms have been electric, but what we have is real.

December 25, 1993

First Christmas I haven't had to concentrate on getting the turkey in the oven at the right time and the potatoes and carrots and dressing and gravy prepared and cooked and on the table, with hot turkey and cranberry and apple-sauce all at the same time. All of this with wrapping last-minute presents and decorating the table. Still, I felt lost with no preparation and no home full of family. This was as it had to be this year. We drove through snow to Marion and Richard's apartment. Richard, not quite sure of his role as man of the house, and Marion, happy to have us but very

We don't know where he was born.

Legend puts him in a manger,

In a stable, among the cattle.

And that seems right. I mean

If God came down from Heaven

Into Mary's womb and joined us

Here in flesh, wretched, precious

> flesh,

Doomed to crucifixion, if that

Is how it was, then a stable's right.

A room in the Holiday Inn would

> never do.

—Ross Woodman,
"Christmas 1993"

anxious about the meal, welcomed us. Everyone was there. Little Aidan, holding on to everything, climbing the piano better than he could walk on the floor. Paul and Kathryn with adorable Marion Rose [nephew, his wife, and their daughter]. She's just over a year, proud to call her father Mama, proud to sing all the time she eats and bangs her spoon, and proud to hurl vases across the room. David home from Vancouver, long hair and ancient clothes, chuckling quietly. Shelley [niece] fierce in her Victorian skirt and blouse. Our big round family table that I so often decorated as an adolescent was pulled full out with all its leaves. I loved seeing it festive for the next generation.

December 26, 1993

Quiet Boxing Day. Paul, Kathryn, and Marion Rose are coming for dinner. It's his birthday. I wish I had the energy to make a cake, but I don't. Poor Paul, all his life he's had a makeshift birthday cake—lemon pie with candles, muffins with candles, trifle with candles. More important to use the energy for conversation than for making cake.

Trying hard to move into the choices of Cronedom. Amazing how easily I accept that word "crone" now! I used to hate its suggestion of a haggard old, cantankerous old, dangerous old woman. But then I saw in the OED its root is the same as "crown"; its shadow side is an old ewe. Well, so be it. Positively, Cronedom is the peak of femininity. It can be the crowning of my life. I have mothered as consciously as I know how, been a container and a mirror for my students and countless others whom I have loved. Now it is time for me to reconnect with my Virgin self—the *I am* within that is one in herself—the Gypsy in my November initiation dream, the 16-year-old who was so strong in her own Being. I need her physical strength, her self-assurance, her connection to that 5-year-old who delights in life. Cronedom for me is freedom from the complexes that cut off my own voice. These I have worked on for 45 years. I have also done my work on the crossroads where God said No and I had to give up my ego desires to the higher destiny. Now I want to become a surrendered instrument.

> The Crone's title was related to the word *crown*, and she represented the power of the ancient tribal matriarch who made the moral and legal decisions for her subjects and descendants.
>
> —*Barbara Walker*, The Crone

Danger of regression for me when the children are here: Positive Mother would accommodate the whole family in every possible way. They don't know me as Crone, living with the limits that make my life my own. They expect me to speak my mind, but they aren't used to the new boundaries.

Accommodating squelches my Crone. She cannot mature if Mother is attempting to care for children, care for husband, care for publisher, care for mailbox and telephone. Gypsy becomes sullen, silent. Gypsy Virgin dies, falls back into the unconscious. Without her, my light goes out. I have to let her live by her own rules. She never could accept the rules of the collective, however lonely that made her. She and Crone belong together. She is my survivor. All my life, even *in utero*, she was determined to live. Yes, love and live—to love, to be loved, and to live. Interesting, to love, to be loved, to live. These do not necessarily go together. To be loved, to be accepted, to be received do not necessarily go with to live. They should, but if a child has to think about making itself fit to be loved, if its body image, the image it carries into society, is not acceptable to the collective, then whoever is living inside that body has to do something extra to make itself acceptable in order to be loved. Given my capacity to love, I suppose I overcompensated in order to be acceptable and lovable.

I think I have done it almost to death's door. In becoming Virgin—who I am, what I believe, what I value, what I live for—I have dared to put most of what I believe into the collective. That is taking a risk. What made me vulnerable was my conviction that what I wanted—consciousness—was what the rest of the world wanted. Was I wrong! Was I wrong all my life! My values are not group values. I donned my social mask and my fat or anorexic social protection, and hoped to survive. Instead of fighting, I acquiesced. Several times, the collision almost brought me to my death. Killed in my own womb.

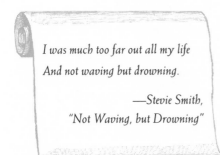

I was much too far out all my life
And not waving but drowning.

—*Stevie Smith,*
"Not Waving, but Drowning"

I look at this photograph of Barry and me sitting on top of the *Scythia* on our way home to Canada in '53, forty years ago. I didn't know Barry; we were

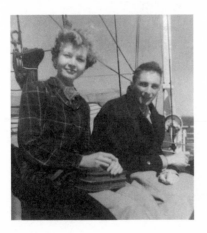

strangers bonded in our fear of returning home. My gypsy had found her freedom rucksacking her way with Mary [deceased friend] through the British Isles and the Continent. There I am on that ship now returning, having to return, knowing I am returning to the place of my failure—my inability to live my own life. But how could I be happy if my family were in pain, trapped in the old patterns? I could not accept happiness outside pain. I knew that going back was returning to my silent prison. I knew I could not hold on to what I had achieved. And yet I could not stop myself. My reality was at home, in that failure, and I had to work myself through that failure detail by detail in order to be truly free. I see the acquiescence in my face, the allowing the ship to carry me home because that was as it had to be.

Now I am once again carried home. Once again fighting for my freedom to live my *I AM*. It lies in day-to-day decisions. It would be so easy to slip into being cared for and caring for Ross. I could quickly become a housemaid, compulsively cleaning and organizing, cooking three meals a day, washing up, and sleeping. My crocodile sleeps so happily. No, I will hold the tension of the opposites right here on Sydenham Street. The long hall is our Highway 401, the distance between his study and mine. To hold the distance and the intimacy at the same time—that is my task. The consciousness I have worked so hard to achieve is at stake.

Dear God, fill my Warrior with strength. Help me to discern which details are of no consequence and which are worth fighting for. Oh, let me handle my sword with love.

Dear Paul, it's sugarless apple crumble with candles for your birthday. How your eyes would twinkle if you knew how I arrived at this conclusion!

> Discriminate:
> passing disturbance;
> soul essence.

December 29, 1993

Trying to be consistent about my herbs. Some dear lady whom I don't know sent me red raspberry leaves to make tea that would comfort my womb. Indeed, it brought fullness to that emptiness. Also echinacea and bags of kelp. And stinging nettles to protect my hair. How very sweet people are! Julian's "sweet touchings of grace."

Also consistent about my afternoon sleep and eight glasses of water. Fully rested for tonight's crowning event.

Last January, out of the blue, a letter arrived saying that Ross would be presented with "a distinguished scholar award" by the Keats-Shelley division of the Modern Languages Association. The date would be December 29, the place the Sheraton Hotel in Toronto. A genuine letting go happened after that letter arrived. A new self-confidence came in.

11:00 P.M.

Tonight was bitter cold. Ross was very handsome in his dark suit and white shirt. His skin had the radiance of a man who has come into his full maturity, rich and full, satisfied with what he has accomplished, and who he is. This night he would be recognized and honored by his academy.

> I will not cease from Mental Fight,
> Nor shall my Sword sleep in my hand,
> Till we have built Jerusalem
> In England's green & pleasant Land.
>
> —William Blake, Milton

Our table was mostly Western [University of Western Ontario] profs—Bal and Chandra, Tillotoma, David, Douglas. In the midst of the elegant meal, Ross became edgy about the lectern—the perennial problem: no lectern. The waiters had to pull up the carpet and shift things radically. But Ross was right: There had to be a microphone and a lectern in order to give dignity and focus to the speeches. So, instead of an old boys' party with old drinkers congratulating one of their own for what he had achieved in life, the brightest Western has to offer gave an astonishing résumé and interpretation of Ross's work. Tillotoma was brilliant in content and style. (She would never have been heard without a microphone.) Ross's response was equally stunning. (Hours of preparation had gone into it.) Douglas was also excellent. Ross shone brightly in his galaxy. It was the climax and letting go of the tension that was never quite resolved during and after his retirement.

As we came home in the taxi, we were proud and punchy.

December 30, 1993

Need to think further into the relationship between matter and psyche in order to work at a deeper level with the imagery. I see the diagrams I used to put on the board.

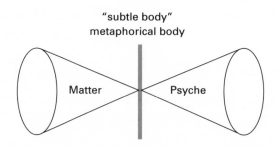

Jung's concept of the cones of energy, matter and psyche, whose apexes touch and do not touch. They "touch" because in the "space" between, body chemistry transforms into imagery, and/or imagery transforms into body chem-

Einstein: $E=mc^2$

istry. They "do not touch" because when Jung wrote this in 1954, psychoneuroimmunology was unknown and the interchange of energies remained a mystery.

My dark images are related to depression as surely as my cancer is related to dark imagery. The connecting space is "the subtle body," the home of metaphor, the world of soul. That's where I'm working now, visualizing radiant energy transforming into healthy cells. Jung knew psyche and matter were not opposites. I know when I speak the poetry I love, energy quickens my cells. My body comes alive. I also know that when Ross was so ill after his retirement from teaching English literature for 42 years, retirement from his beloved classroom and poetry, he happened into Jeanne Achterberg's imagery workshop in Esalen. In one hour, a "Pulsation of the Artery," he found his images again and was on his way back to wholeness. This is subtle body work—attunement to a new vibration.

There is a corner I am trying to contact. It is that tiny voice in my body that says, "I can't." It's that tiny possum in me that senses abandonment or rejection in the atmosphere, becomes petrified with fear, and stays absolutely still in order to survive. That is my survivor; it is also my despair. That's the corner I need to fill with transformative light. That despair began *in utero,* the daughter who was not a son. Paradoxically, that terror of being abandoned is the very gasoline that has driven me all my life. Now I no longer need to fear, or to be driven.

I see another diagram.

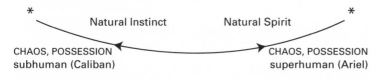

*   Natural Instinct   Natural Spirit   *

CHAOS, POSSESSION
subhuman (Caliban)
                     CHAOS, POSSESSION
superhuman (Ariel)

I see the pendulum of energy swinging rhythmically between the instinctual and spiritual poles. Then it gains momentum because I am overtired. It begins to swing too far toward the spiritual side. I am no longer interested in food or rest or responsibility. I want music, poetry, prayer, freedom. I am Ariel. Gradually the compensatory swing takes me beyond the normal instinctual pole into bodily Caliban cravings—driven body desires or blank inertia. Ariel is a spirit; Caliban is an abandoned creature, part human, part beast; both are possessed. In this addictive swing, the pendulum is out of kilter. It swings outside the boundaries of the human poles into chaotic behavior on both sides. The upshot on one side is an imagination charged with death imagery; on the other, physical exhaustion—beyond the beyond.

My dreams and I are working on a new harmonic for our orchestra. I need to rest without any agenda for at least a year. Just relax into safekeeping and allow the new imagery to come into my cells. Even to think that thought

PROS. (TO ARIEL): My tricksy spirit! . . .

PROS. (TO CALIBAN): . . . and this

     demidevil

. . . this thing of darkness I

Acknowledge mine.

     —*Shakespeare,* The Tempest

connects me to that dark hole in my body that can become catatonic with fear. Sophia can pierce that fear. She turns "I can't" into "Let's try. New life is possible. I bore you through India. I helped you to understand, 'Death once dead, there's no more dying then'" (Shakespeare, Sonnet 146).

Another rung of the spiral. I am letting go of fear. I am increasingly open to the love in the golden web. I am experiencing death as birth, as passage into a new frequency.

December 31, 1993

Drove back to London after sessions with Zeca and Helga. Always feel nourished and seen and heard with both of them. The 401 was filthy and ferocious with immense trucks. Stopped at McDonald's for Ross's McChicken and my McMuffin (though I prefer Tim Horton's).

Cozy afternoon preparing for our annual New Year's Eve celebration with John and Mary. Phone calls from Eileen, Sandra, Paula, Carolyn, Bruce and Cherry. Arranged flowers and white candles. House fragrant with hyacinth and narcissus from Barbara and Catherine.

John carried in our perennial salmon. When he was stretched out on the floor beside the fire, he was perfectly happy. The four of us talked straight from the bone about where our lives are and where we hope they might be going. None of us feared risking honesty. Rare relationship!

January 1, 1994

Annual New Year's pancakes with Robert and Marguerite and their young sons. Warm afterglow of Christmas tree and cards, at the same time anticipating new life.

Spent the afternoon in bed watching the New Year's program from Vienna. Memories '53. La la la ♪ ♪lalala ♪♪la la la! Alfred and lilacs, waltzing and wine and Alfred, Mozart cakes and Alfred, "singer boys" and white stallions and Alfred. "Loveliest of Latin teachers," he whispered, as he kissed my "beautiful hand" good-bye.

Somewhat overwhelming looking ahead to that vast expanse of unknown, uncharted territory, wondering where next December 31 will find us. That's a very real question, Ross being 71 and I 65 with cancer now a part of our lives.

That time of year thou mayst
*   in me behold*
When yellow leaves, or
*   none, or few, do hang*
Upon those boughs which
*   shake against the cold,*
Bare ruin'd choirs, where
*   late the sweet birds sang.*

—*Shakespeare, Sonnet 73*

January 4, 1994

Concentrating on my schedule, trying to keep focused on one hour's rest at noon, food, supplements.

Vitamin and Food Recommendations from Stephan Rechtschaffen,
*   M.D., to me*
(to be used with Ultra-Clear Sustain)

1. Multivitamin—Thorne—high-potency multivitamin—3–6 per day.

2. None or very little iron—iron is an oxidant—oxidation goes on in chemical process—oxidation causes little burns on cellular levels. Body protects with antioxidants—vitamins A, E, C; selenium.
3. Vitamin E 400 IU—1 per day.
4. Vitamin C—2000 mg—3 times per day—builds immune system.
5. Echinacea—3 per day—supports immune system.
6. Thymus-based T-cell (thymus cell)—2 or 3 per day—encourage thymus by beating my chest. Image Sophia. Take her through my whole body.
7. EPA from cold-water fish—1 capsule 3x per day.
8. Cod-liver oil—1 tablespoon.
9. Thorne—pure antioxidant formula—1 or 2 per day.
10. Diet: eliminate red meat, fried foods, fat, caffeine. Stay with fresh green and yellow vegetables (the greener and yellower the better). Garlic.
11. Herbal teas, green teas, essiac.

Also concentrating on my psychic focus:

1. Keep asking questions. Don't allow myself to fall into passive response.
2. Act from my own feeling. What is the real value here? Stay with that and act on it. I have a role in this healing with the medical world as well as the naturopathic.

Our task would seem to lie in being able successfully to demonstrate somatic events as part of a correlated psychosomatic total evolution, and in finding the dynamic categories or laws which represent the common elements of these complementary psychic and physical evolutions. In short, we are looking for a "generalized field theory" of psychosomatics.

—*Edward C. Whitmont,*
Psyche and Substance

3. Accept maximum medical care.
4. Accept maximum homeopathic care.
5. Check parameters of safety re: radiation.
6. Dance. Let the other side come to me.
7. Walk in fresh air. Breathe deeply. Sing as I walk.
8. Prayer, meditation, visualization, anytime, day or night.
9. Check out any negative attitudes. Go for the positive.
10. Cleansing body, cleansing mind.

January 8, 1994

Somewhere in these first days of January, I went to the court of inquiry for Fraser's estate. Spent two days going through sheaves of papers clarifying dates and exact details. Took my "training" for three hours the day before and was "grilled" for five hours in the actual sessions. Some of the legal training was good medical training: "Listen to the exact question. Do not answer more than the question asks. Do not be afraid to say, 'I don't know.' Answer as truthfully as you can."

It went quite well. I am trying now to make the decisions that will clarify my will and testament.

> No bird soars too high, if he soars with his own wings.
>
> —William Blake,
> "The Marriage of Heaven and Hell"

January 11, 1994

Mother, your birthday. And Sir John A.'s [Macdonald, first prime minister of Canada]. I light the candle for your 94th birthday, wherever you are.

Mother, you gave me life in your death. "Be free," you said. I'm trying to live the freedom you lived and died to give me. The greatest gift you could have given, Mother Dear.

Let me not be sentimental. I am your daughter; I know *genuine* feeling. To keep my choices clear, I carry a scrap of paper in my wallet. Do you remember how, when your memory began to fail, you used to phone to ask me for quotations you loved? You wrote them down. I didn't know it then, but I know now; you pinned them to your petticoat so they were part of you.

When you died in St. Jo's, while I was rushing home from Zurich, I was devastated. Ross and I went to your apartment the next day. A scrap of paper lay on the table. Did you know, Mother? Did you leave it there for me? Were you cutting the cord you knew I could not cut? In your beautiful handwriting,

> And whether we shall meet again I know not.
> Therefore our everlasting farewell take:
> For ever, and for ever, farewell, Cassius!
> If we do meet again, why, we shall smile;
> If not, why then, this parting was well made.

> (Shakespeare, *Julius Caesar*)

I wanted you to die my way. God had another way. Mother, teach me now as you taught me then to surrender my ego desires to God. Smile on me as I begin at the clinic today. Forever, Marnie.

Got up early. Visualization, bringing golden light through my fingers into my womb area, relishing the roundness of my body. Feeling the gold turn into purple and pulsing through my every cell.

Nervous that the car won't start in the cold, nervous about driving to the hospital in the snow. Began preparations at seven to be at the hospital by nine. No problems with the Toyota or the snow. Steady, stoic drive! People friendly at the clinic. The young technician came to me with three large paper cups of "orange juice" and said, "Drink one of those in each of the following twenty minutes." Watched children playing and drank until I was bloated. Went to post my letters at 10:15, returned to find the staff ready for me. Put on blue pajama pants and loose top, drank another ten ounces of "orange juice," asked the young man what exactly this machine was measuring.

"Don't you know what you're here for?" he barked.

"I don't need a put-down, young man," I said quietly. "I'm far enough down already."

He came to his senses and explained that the CAT scan would pick up any unusual formation in the abdomen (where they were going to work). I asked if it would pick up cancer.

"Unusual cell formations," he said, evading my question.

Anyway, the room was beautiful, backlit cream, paintings by Canadians on the walls, and the big cream machine in the middle.

"The bed moves. The machine moves," he said. "Just breathe and let go when I tell you. Absolute stillness."

I lay absolutely still on his order and released on his order. Twenty minutes, and I was finished, thankful to God that I live in Canada and have been paying Ontario Health Insurance Plan since its inception in 1950. All this care I deserve.

Lost my way home. Found myself driving through fields of white snow, ended up in Nilestown. Couldn't do any-

> Every time we say "your will be done" we should have in mind all possible misfortunes added together.
>
> —*Simone Weil*

thing but try to find Hamilton Road. Got home about 11:30. Realized my Toronto women's group was right then saying healing prayers for me. Felt terribly sick. Body collapsed before I got my green coat off. Too weak to get it off and too cold. Went to bed in boots and coat and opened myself to their prayers. Felt the love pouring into my cells, felt them releasing me into taking responsibility for my own healing process. Certainly there was a shift. Opened totally, wept, and went to sleep. Awoke about three, took off coat, boots, clothes, and got under warm covers. So very tired.

Couldn't watch TV. The violence, the teenagers mindlessly destroying and killing, is too much. I become desperate and my body becomes rigid. A gang broke into our parking basement while we were away at Christmas and broke the windows in sixteen cars. Took nothing but one quarter left in a car for parking.

My bulbs in the kitchen are growing. A veritable garden there. Two cyclamen in full bloom, crocuses coming, white narcissus, hyacinths, tulips, and daffodils, dancing in the sun. Bruce's spring pot arrived.

Bruce [brother] is pulling back energy for himself now. After 25 years of television he is going to go on the stage again—big part in a play that may reach the West End. He got what he wanted, the part and second billing, and I think he wonders now what he is doing. At 63 the memory work is hard, and each day they are rewriting and reblocking—as they will be while the play is on the road. He says he feels the tightness in his chest. He hadn't thought about the physical energies required for traveling and for working in a different theater every two weeks. He likes the part and the creative energy required. I hope his body can take it.

So all this goes on and Ross is on an art consultant's trip to New York. Tonight he goes to *Angels in America*. It's billed as the play that gives the stage a new direction for the new millennium. Tony Kushner is the author. It strikes into the nineties' morality crises, the AIDS crisis, corruption in leadership, *perestroika* in America. All sounds very serious, but it's done in camp style with an acrobatic angel as a messenger from on high announcing, "The Great Work Begins." I'd just like to see if she's a Sacred Prostitute announcing to the godforsaken world and even godforsaken heaven that The Great Work that is beginning is the realization of the feminine as the bridge between God and humankind. That's what the Sacred Prostitute was in the past. Her body was holy, and through her body men found the eros that connected them to God. In recognizing her body as sacred, they recognized their own body as sacred, and experienced the one world as sacred. That's The Great Work that's beginning. But I'm not sure that's what *Angels in America* is about.

Remarkable how God organizes our lives: I pray that He will help me to bring my Spiritual Warrior to conscious-

I will rise now, and go about the city in the streets, and in the broadways I will seek him whom my soul loveth: I sought him, but I found him not.

—*The Song of Solomon III, 2*

Someday after mastering the winds, the waves, the tides and gravity, we shall harness for God the energies of love, and then for the second time in the history of the world, man will discover fire.

—*Teilhard de Chardin*

ness; He hears me, and He moves Ross off to New York so that I have to muster every ounce of Spiritual Warrior in myself to defend my feminine feelings and values. No projections allowed!

January 12, 1994

Drove to clinic to have tattooing done—the stenciling that will tell the technicians exactly where the radiation will go. Still uncertain about doing radiation at all. Yesterday I felt it was all unnecessary. If I worked with Zeca and Helga, took the essiac, took the live cell therapy and the multivitamins, perhaps I would be basically clear of cancer cells in a few weeks. But then I remember how well I felt when my womb was full of cancer, then I lose faith in my own relationship to my own body. When I was anorexic, I always felt that starvation brought me close to God. It brought me close to death, a Demon Lover, whose radiance lured my senses into a life so exquisite I yearned to escape gross matter. That Demon is swinging on the pendulum with the Death Goddess, who would silently enclose me in her arms. I fear them. I fear the silent killers. I fear I could be walking straight into death without knowing it. I've almost done it several times before. I've known addicts who were lured into their own trap and slipped over with-

Faced with the precarious existence of tribal life—drought, sickness, evil influences—the shaman responded by ridding his body of weight and flying to another world, another level of perception, where he could find the strength to change the face of reality.

—*Italo Calvino,*
Six Memos for the Next Millenium

out knowing they were leaving this reality until it was too late to pull back.

Well, I waited at the clinic. There were Christmas cookies and coffee on the table—neither of which I am supposed to have. But I enjoyed BOTH. Eventually, Mrs. Woodman was called. For the stenciling I went into a backlit room, handsome cream machine, and paintings on the wall. I lay down on the little cot; four fairylike creatures whisked around me in delicate white dresses. (I was glad they weren't in mauve and pink crinkled organdy.) They all introduced themselves to make me feel recognized and at home. No doctor in sight. A big machine on the ceiling was ready to do its work. They put my torso in exact position and all disappeared. A voice from another world said, "Hold your breath—absolutely still." Whirring noises began and the machine changed colors in specific slots and a beam burned red. Whisk—and my four fairies were in again, fixing me this way and that to get the exact marking. I had no complaints. "Be as compulsive as you wish," I thought. "I enjoy your perfection. Be perfect. Oh, be perfect. Don't let the radiation go one-sixteenth of an inch into my bowel or my bladder. Oh, please, Sophia, let them be perfect."

Then my soul got out on the ceiling. She sat up there quite quiet and not angry with me.

"I'm doing what I have to do to live," I said to her.

"Yes," she sadly agreed. "Are you sure you need to go through

. . . [B]elief in the scriptures is literally the act of turning one's own body inside-out—imagining, creating, the capacity for symbolic and religious thought begin with the capacity to endow interior physical events with an external, nonphysical referent.

—*Elaine Scarry,*
The Body in Pain

this burning? Do you think there is any cancer left that we couldn't get rid of if we visualized enough?"

"I don't know," I said. "I can't think anymore."

Then my body wanted to vomit and shit, and wanted off that bed. "I'm not going to stay here," she said. "You know better than to bring me here, Marion. How could you set me up for this scorching? I've cared for you all your life. I've compensated. I'll do it again if you give me rest and proper food. I've taken you where you were supposed to go when God wanted to move you. I got you out of the womb you went back to in Forest High School. I got you out of South Secondary School, and before that I got you to India. Now I can't understand why you don't realize that the dead baby in your womb has been removed and we are ready to go on to new life. If you damage me—my immune system is already in trouble—what will become of us?"

"It's all true," I said. "It's all true. You've been a wonderful body. God has repeatedly spoken to me through you. Picked me up by the scruff of my neck and the seat of my pants and forcibly removed me from a dead situation and forced me into a new. But cancer is different. I did not detect it in October and I'm not sure I can now. There is a loophole in my psyche that I could slip through into death."

And all the time this three-way conversation is going on, I'm thinking, "Why is this taking so long? Are they finding more cancer? Why are they moving the machine up so far on my chest? What is wrong? Cancer in my lungs? It's metastasized. I'm going to die. Marion, you're going to die!"

Then the four fairies came swishing in and put marks on my outer thigh where the terrible pain had been in my leg.

"Lymph," I thought. "It's in the lymph. That's been the real trouble all along. We never looked beyond the uterus. It's all through me."

Then my doctor came skipping in. He was scrutinizing my film. "I've found something in your liver," he said.

"That's it," I thought. "Rosie [friend] had liver cancer. She lived six weeks or less. I'll not take the radiation. I'll live six weeks as I want to live—not burn myself up." I sat up and said to him, "Are you telling me I have cancer in the liver?"

"No," he said. "But there is something nobody else found in your liver. Could be cancer, could be a cyst, could be a fat deposit."

My body decided she was getting out of there fast. I was trying to get off the bed. I could feel the diarrhea assembling itself for a real onslaught.

Maybe the doctor saw the frozen terror in my eyes. "You'd better go to ultrasound now," he said, "if they're still open."

The clock said four. "For sure they'll be closed," I thought.

I walked through miles of corridors to where I was yesterday. Yes, they were open. Yes, the technician was waiting for me. I put on the blue pajamas, lay down, and she began rubbing the firm ball under my right breast, pushing hard. I was sure I'd hear a long beep. I thought a beep might tell her where the cancer was. I kept watching her eyes, just to be sure she didn't pretend there was nothing there so she could get the doctor to tell me the truth—the older doctor, Dr. MacMillan, who came and said who he was, "just so you won't think I am an intruding presence who happened to wander in."

"No, I watched you while I was drinking my 'orange juice' yesterday," I said. " I know you're a doctor. I trust you."

So together they worked. "Can't pick up anything," he said. Then he phoned for the CAT scan to be brought over.

Another fifteen minutes, during which I decided if I was going to die, it was all right. Just have to adjust the focus. I realized that Ross and I are living with Death as a daily ally. Death is right here. "If it be now, 'tis not to come; if it be not to come, it will be now; if it be not now, yet it will come: the readiness is all" (*Hamlet*).

"The readiness is all," as I had written on my ironic notification card last September. I believe Jung's idea that the body carries the conflict that the psyche cannot consciously endure. In my situation, I knew the summons my body was carrying. I also knew the summons my psyche was carrying. But I was not ready to obey God's calendar instead of my own.

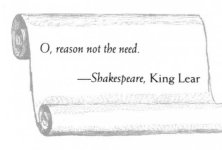

O, reason not the need.

—*Shakespeare*, King Lear

So all this thinking is going on while I lie freezing and shaking on the bed beside the ultrasound machine. Finally the kind old doctor returned and said he had seen the CAT scan. Yes, it was true there was something in the liver. And bless them, he and the technician stayed until six trying to find exactly where it was. They didn't send me home in agony and say, "Come back at two on Friday—or next week." Finally he said, "There may be a cyst there. There may be a fat deposit—maybe something you were born with. But don't worry about it. We can't find it; things like this are common."

Somehow his calm and experience gave me peace. I got dressed, feeling I had escaped the gallows once more, and skipped through the corridors like a 16-year-old and into the snowy, dark

Yet somewhere in these years

the heart set out to break,

feet climbed beyond the bounds,

began the climb.

—*Tom Yeomans*, Soul Canticles

parking lot and drove home. No Nilestown detour this time. My brains were right there.

But I went instantly to bed. Felt like I used to feel in India when I'd escaped black-market money buyers, desperate tradesmen grabbing my arms, poor, blind, crippled beggars on the ground and dozens of children tearing at my dress. I'd finally get into my room and shut the door and fall into bed or onto the floor. India too was a powerful initiation.

January 13, 1994

Took my spring flowers to Heather. She reminded me that Sylvia had cancer twice and is still alive. I love to hear about the survivors.

Slept on the bus to Toronto. Spent too much energy trying to find a post office in the Eaton Centre, but I wanted to get some mail weighed and off—and did. Then to the studio. Felt so safe in my mauves and burgundies on the seventeenth floor.

Then read a magazine article that someone had sent me. It was about a person's embarrassment when he lived on after people thought he would be dead. They had put everything on to him, loved him, treasured him because he was going to die. They projected their love of their own departure from this world on to him. He didn't depart, and nobody wanted him when he came back into life. What kind of encouragement is that supposed to be? From a friend! A joke?

> Nothing is more punitive than to give a disease a meaning—that meaning being invariably a moralistic one. . . . The disease itself becomes a metaphor.
>
> —*Susan Sontag*, Illness as Metaphor

Projections! Projections! "It's the father complex, kills the mother, tears out her womb." Or "It's the Negative Mother imprinted on your cells driving you to death." Or "Endometrial cancer is found to have a hereditary factor." Or "You never gave up your grief for Fraser. Your grief is destroying you." Or "Tear things to shreds. Let your rage go." Or "The cancer personality gives all to others and keeps nothing for itself, and when it has given all, it gives more."

I am amazed, astonished at how people dare to psychoanalyze one another when they have no real knowledge of circumstances—external or internal—no knowledge of the dreams, no knowledge of the inner landscape! They throw their own crud on to the one who is sick. Real danger of becoming the scapegoat who takes on the projections and then runs away into the woods carrying others' loads. Or being sacrificed. There it is! There is the person who lives on after others have put their love of death on to him, sacrificed him to their gods. The grand crescendo of love that doesn't move into death but splutters back into life. Unforgivable in an apocalyptic society!

January 14, 1994

Felt very vulnerable with Helga as I told her about my doctor and his take on the possibility of cancer in my liver. I believed him. A month ago I would not have believed, but now I am realizing that I do have cancer and that the cells are virulent, that it is a killer—in its early stages, a silent killer. I have seen enough to know how cruel it is. I could not look into Helga's eyes. That is unusual for me. The terror was incredible. If she or Zeca had said, "Yes, I think you have cancer in your liver," I would have felt the end rising in front of me. Anyway, Helga gave me a remedy to help counteract the radiation, more essiac, and an excellent treatment. Then a treatment from Zeca, some remedies, and reassurance from him that he thought we could be rid of the dangerous cells in a few months. He sees my lack of trust in my own connection to my body. "It is your destiny," he said. "Your life, your death. You must choose. What I can do is support your body through the radiation if you decide to take it."

So once again reassembled, I cuddled into my green Victorian coat and took the subway to Dundas Street. When I got off the train, I sensed someone looking at me. I looked around. Sure enough, eyes inside a hood were looking, intense. I instantly felt it was Cathleen [friend], whom I hadn't seen for at least five years. I was as glad to see her as she to see me, although we've had almost no communication. She helped me with my bag and walked to the bus depot, telling me about finishing her training, her happy marriage, her dancing child, and her happiness in her new work. Then I told her I have cancer, am closing my office, looking forward to writing. We just looked at each other.

She said, " You know, I knew it was you in that space before I saw you."

"And I knew it was you in the hood," I said. (It was exactly the same dynamic that ignited at Eglinton and Yonge the day I was almost blown into the traffic by the wind. She saw that moment and realized how human, how frail I was in contrast to her archetypal image of me.) Anyway, we had a *meeting*. We were both totally present in soul. We looked into each other's eyes and said good-bye as I got on the bus. It was so extraordinary because there was an unhappiness in our parting five years ago, maybe a sense of betrayal on both sides. In the meeting, in the seconds before the actual eye contact, our bodies greeted each other with greatest excitement, like two children running ahead of their parents. Then we met and realized how glad we were to be together again. Then the possibility of forever separation and the full realization of what we were, are, and will always be to each other.

January 16, 1994

So glad to have Ross home. Wonderful tales of New York galleries, ballet, opera. But the theater was it this time: *Angels in America*. The writing and staging were innovative, outrageous, and hilarious. Great theater! As for "The Great Work" to be done, my idea of the angel as Sacred Prostitute seems to be straight idealization. Ross saw a Nietzschean world, a world where there is no god, no sacred book. We are on our own. We have to improvise and do what we can for ourselves. "The Great Work" is the invention of ourselves, even as the play is an invention of ourselves. And as for the angel, she flies on pulleys that we can see, an impoverished homemade creature. So much for that projection! At least I brought to consciousness what I think "The Great Work" is.

I think Ross found it unreal and disorienting being in New York and leaving me home here—especially with cancer. But I need his strength, and I know he has to get away into artistic space to find it. Mr. N. told me his great moment in New York was watching Ross looking at, perceiving Jim Dine's *Cat & Ape*. He sees with his inner eye.

He got into real Woody Allen high jinx that only he could pull off. He, Martin and Ann and Mr. and Mrs. N. were in a stretch limousine trying to get out of the city to Martin's car. Because of the storm, the bridges out of New York were blocked. The journey took five hours, mostly standing in traffic. Ross's diabetes has an unnegotiable effect on his kidneys. Martin took the champagne glasses out of the limo bar, lined them up on the floor, Ross knelt in front of Martin and filled the glasses one after another while Ann and Mr. and Mrs. N. gazed sedately out the window. He told the story with such elegance that Martin and I were crying with laughter.

January 17, 1994

As we watched the 7:30 news this morning, suddenly Bryant Gumbel was saying, "Something wrong, something's trying to come through." A broken, terrified voice came over the wire: the worst earthquake in years in L.A. with epicenter in the San Fernando Valley. I became very tense thinking about Jill, Gina, Nils, Patty, Barbra, Virginia, so many of the women in the workshops. That

The very God! think, Abib; dost
   thou think?
So, the All-Great, were the All-
   Loving too—
So, through the thunder comes a
   human voice,
Saying, "O heart I made, a heart
   beats here!"

   —Robert Browning, "An Epistle"

thought stretched out to all my dear ones in California; they'll be devastated psychologically.

Marea once told me how petrified her body was in the last earthquake. The earth cracking open under her feet, the walls tumbling, objects crashing, no solid ground anywhere. Afterward, in spite of her conscious effort to control her terror, her body animal went into the same paralysis in every aftershock. My little possum silently shouted, "Of course." I understood "ground" in a new way. Spent most of the day in bed, watching, praying for my friends.

Terribly cold—minus 46 degrees with the wind chill factor. Thinking that bursting pipes and a motor that won't go are nothing compared to what is going on in L.A. Ross and I went shopping, and I ran over to the postbox, less than half a block away. It was so cold I felt my face stiffening and my hand barely able to hold the mail. Half a block! I've never experienced cold like that except in Timmins and there we were dressed in long johns and overstockings. Came home and didn't try to go out again all week. Worried about the stale air in the house. The books say I must breathe fresh air in long, deep breaths into my belly and I must drink eight glasses of water a day. Not tea, not coffee, not juice, or even lemon water in that eight glasses. Eight glasses of water. And fresh air. Cancer cells cannot live in oxygen. In spite of that knowledge, I did not want that bone cold settling in my body, so I did not go out until Sunday.

The windows were magic. As I talked to Deanne on the phone in the kitchen, smelling my hyacinths and narcissus, I watched the frost creating Japanese pictures—plants, ferns, mountains veiled in mist. Haven't seen that since I was a kid—Jack Frost painting on the panes. He was invisible, so was his brush, but there, before my eyes, his images appeared, "Clothed in white samite, mystic, wonderful" (Tennyson, *Idylls of the King*).

Pauline [doctor friend] phoned. She helped me with the positive side of radiation. When I told her about the spacious rooms and the paintings and the splendid, yes, beautiful machines and how hard the technicians worked to please my doctor, she said, "'Almost thou persuadest me . . .' This doctor is a perfectionist, Marion. One-sixteenth of an inch—that's all that matters to you from him. The more compulsive he is, the better. Let him and his technicians take as long as they want to make everything exact. So he isn't sensitive, doesn't believe in soul? If he can run that machine perfectly, that's fine."

I think of everything I've ever written about perfection and death. Here it is in spades. The perfection of the machine. My soul and my body in the power of that machine and the perfectionist mind that controls it. When I said to my doctor that I believed radiation could cause cancer, he agreed. When I asked, "Where does the creative side of radiation begin?" he was silent for a moment. Then he said fiercely, "There is no creative side. It is all destruction. We are here to kill virulent cells. Virulence versus virulence." I am glad to know exactly where he stands. It is a relief not to have to expect anything from him except the perfection of his technology. That I do expect.

Talked to Pauline again as the tension grew around radiation. "You know," she said, "idealization can be a lack of femininity. If you idealize to the point of blinding yourself to what may save your life, that is not being on the side of life, the positive side of the feminine. Blindness is negative."

"Yes. Othello killed his beloved soul for the cause," I said. "Idealization is part of the perfection that kills. We are living in 1994. Science and technology need not be the driven masculine. Radiant masculinity can be the creative masculine spirit radiating through the density of the nega-

> The result of all this [addiction to perfection] is that we are no longer born. We begin as surgical extractions and we end as surgical extinctions. Between the beginning and the end we are a chemically operated machine subject to more and more refined technology.
>
> —*Marion Woodman*,
> Addiction to Perfection

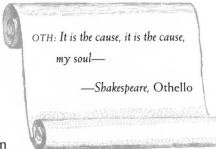

OTH: *It is the cause, it is the cause, my soul—*

—*Shakespeare*, Othello

tive mother concretized in cancer. Surely there is a way spirit and nature can come together. Surely I can use Sophia's shield to block the dangerous rays, open myself to healing. Trust the process day to day."

Pauline agreed. The decision is mine. We talked about women caught in idealization when they are determined to bear a child artificially and give themselves over to drugs month after month. Doctors now know that some of those drugs cause cancer. Still, we have to look at each case individually to see what is negative, what is positive. Then I feel my poor body. So sweet, so innocent, so courageous!

January 24, 1994

7:30 A.M.

In one hour Tom will arrive to take me to the clinic for my first radiation. Dear Sophia, go with me. Please know that I am not doing this without anguish. I would not injure your earth in any way if I could help it. On some level, I still believe I could heal myself. But medical science says it can give me a 98 percent chance of life after cancer. I do not believe I am to die yet. So I am doing this horrendous thing. Please be with me. Please be my shield. Shield out all that is not necessary to my healing. And please allow me to be open to the radiance that can heal me. Help me to be open to what is creative, closed to what is destructive. Into thy loving arms I commend my spirit. Keep me open to process. Be very close to me every minute. Let me know what to do spontaneously. Tell me if I should stop. Let me not be trapped in a conventional treatment that lasts five times a week for five weeks with forty-eight hours' holocaust at the end. Let me move with it daily, in the moment.

I love your sacred earth, in which I live, move, and have my Being. I love you. Into thy hands I commend my bodysoul. She is frightened. Please help me to love her into knowing this is for her continuing life. This is not instinct. This is not nature. No, this is science working with nature to open up new possibilities.

Dear Sophia, hold your daughter in your arms.

2:00 P.M.

Tom arrived at 8:30 with a pot of purple crocuses. Spring is coming. As I went out to get into his car, five Canadian geese went squawking overhead right above us. Both of us opened our arms, ran to each other, and said, "The gods are propitious." Having decided to do this, I was not nervous or halting. I simply went forward to do what seemed necessary in order to be free to live.

Sarah gave me my five-day-a-week-for-five-weeks timetable, told me to bring it back every day. I went in, lay down on the bed. The doctor said they would all be going out of the room. "Lie still and breathe normally." Two Chinese young men put my body in exact position and went out. I waited, heard a buzzing like a buzz saw for fifteen seconds, then a higher buzz for five. Shut down. The men came in, rolled the machine under me, out, again the twenty seconds. Again they reentered, rolled the machine to the left side of my hip, out, again the buzz. Again they reentered, rolled it to the right hip, out, twenty-second buzz, and it was over. They assured me it would take less time tomorrow because they would not have to do their calculations. I asked one if they could identify cancer cells with a CAT scan. "No," he said. "The CAT scan identifies irregularities, but the 'irregularities' have to be put under a microscope to find out if they are cancer and what kind." It took me so long to find that out because my question was not exact enough.

So, feeling a bit scrambled, I found Tom, and we came home talking about the dangers of putting up twelve high-rises near the Sifton Bog.

Felt very shaky as I peeled my yellow vegetables for lunch. Prepared them, but couldn't eat them. Too tired. Too totally out of it. Today it all seems too much. Ross and I were at Sydenham yesterday. It seemed huge, filthy, exposed, far too open to the street on all sides—and so much to be done. It was good to come back to our little womb world, hidden away from the eyes of everyone.

This cara weeseed, Pretty mites, my sweetthings, was they poor-loves abandoned by wholawidey world?

—*James Joyce*, Finnegans Wake

Now my throat is getting sore, a lot of mucus, my voice deepening by the moment. Thank God, I did that heavy, strict, Ultra-Clear Sustain metabolic clearing cleanse over a week ago. That gave me deep fatigue and choking mucus. Obviously, a big cleanse was necessary, and now a bigger one with the radiation.

Bruce sent another mystical bouquet—three smaller ginger flowers, pink carnations, mauve daisies.

Dr. Cohen phoned. I asked her if it was true that radiation can produce cancer ten or fifteen years down the road. "Yes," she said, "certain types of cancer, but the chances are slim. The radiation goes for the cells that divide quickly and are therefore highly sensitive to radiation. Cancer cells divide more quickly than most normal cells. But the cells in the inside lining of bowel and bladder are especially sensitive to radiation because they too divide quickly. Long term, these cells can create problems like bladder irritation or narrowing of the rectum or chronic diarrhea." Well, I'll take the remedies, and do the best I can for my immune system by bringing in light energy through imagery.

Talked to Frances just now. She has three hyacinths sitting in the sunshine in her kitchen. She waters my soul every morning as she waters them.

Ross asked me to go over some mail with him. I was looking at him, knowing I should answer, and fell asleep with my eyes open. Strong stuff they're giving me! Too strong.

David M. phoned tonight, David K. on Sunday, David B., David C.—these so-important Davids in our lives. Also Robert, Greg, and Bill. If people's love can make me well, I will be blooming with health. The inner work is my own.

January 25, 1994

Tom and I at 8:30—our motto: *Five wild geese fly free and honking*. Tom told me about a tape by Kathleen Battle and Jessye Norman—spirituals. "There Is a Balm in Gilead." I have to find that tape. Just to hear those words made my flesh hum. Somewhere there is a deep sadness in me—sadness for the world, for children, for adolescents. Nothing is free of chaos. That grief is in me, and I know I won't be free of cancer if I can't let that sadness pass through me. There is something about Blacks singing Blues that makes sense to me. Sing it like it is, in all its horror. Let the body move, clap, roar it out, cry it out, shout it out, fall on the floor weep it out—but face it like it is and let it go.

Ross and I went shopping for groceries at Loblaws. So much garbage on the shelves. Boxes, bottles, plastics, junk food, junk, junk, junk. Part of me wants to run outside the minute I go in. But I know we can discriminate and buy what we need. I have to keep going to Loblaws. I know I had a phobia about this in September. When I thought of going I couldn't be bothered.

January 26, 1994

Seems incredible. I've been to the clinic only three times. Tom arrived in great spirits. One of his crocuses had bloomed overnight in my kitchen—rich dark purple. Fantastic how an ugly bulb carries within it the archetypal field that produces that particular leaf, flower, color. The big amaryllis bulb is also in full glory. Four red bells on one stock and two out and two ready to burst on the other. A miracle, millions of miracles, we rarely notice. As Tom and I grieved over the Sifton Bog, we could almost hear the monstrous iron fingers pulling out the earth for the twelve ugly high-rises that will give some developer more money.

And with that we arrived at the clinic. They're getting to know me now. Everyone is all smiles. Surely they don't dare think what they are doing to life. I don't believe it can be right. Had my checkup with a nurse, Ann-Marie. Very sweet, she was. When I told her how tired I am, she said she suspected I must have an underlying depression. The side effects should not be showing up yet. I decided to test her out before I said too much.

"How can I release the radiation toxins from my body?" I asked. "I'm taking lemon juice and peel, essiac, lecithin."

"We don't suggest you take any citrus juices or fruits," she said. "And no raw vegetables or juices, no broccoli, cabbage, sprouts, cauliflower, turnip, no fiber. There's danger of chronic diarrhea. Stay away from anything that will cause gas. But you shouldn't be feeling any of this yet."

"Well, I am," I said. "I'm full of gas all the time and hourly running to the bathroom."

"You shouldn't be doing that yet," she said. "Eat a bland diet. Anything you want—bland meat with no spices . . ."

"So much for my steamed green and yellow vegetables," I thought, knowing I was going to continue to eat them, gas or no gas. I have nothing else.

"Maybe you should see the social worker," she said.

"What can she do for me?" I asked.

"She can help you with financial difficulties."

"That's not one of my worries," I said.

"Your marital problems. I notice your husband doesn't bring you."

"I need my husband to be strong at home." I said. "He is too sensitive to this environment. His body takes in the despair and death and terror that pulse within these walls and then both of us have to deal with that when we go home. My friend is happy to bring me. He's sensitive too, but I'm not his soul mate in danger of dying."

The veils started to fall over her eyes. "Perhaps you need a community support system," she said.

"I have many friends," I said. "I am not lonely."

"Then why are you depressed?" she said, her voice trembling with irritation because she couldn't seem to help me—no, because I wouldn't receive her help.

"I am depressed, " I said, "because I feel I am betraying the Great Mother. She loves me. She has given me this sacred body to cherish. I am allowing it to be bombed with atomic bombs, just the way Hiroshima was bombed. The technicians set those tiny crosses in those tiny holes to match the tiny circles tattooed on my body, and they're perfect gunners. Thank God they are! I hope they never hit my bowel or my bladder. One-sixteenth of an inch too deep or too broad and I'm in trouble for the rest of my life. Of course, I'm depressed. I HATE everything that's being done to me here. But I want to live."

That did it. Her eyes glazed. "You'd better talk to the social worker," she said.

"I know I'm not being a cooperative patient," I said. "Statistics say cooperative patients don't do as well as uncooperative ones. I'm not attacking you. I'm trying to find my soul. I think she's up on the ceiling watching. She's not angry; she's not defeated. She's guarding."

As I began to open up, I could see Ann-Marie closing her notebook and taking off her glasses. Shades of the London establishment that drove me to Zurich in 1974. If I spoke my mind, I was written off as a lost cause. So I got up, thanked her, and found the technicians waiting outside the door for me. Once again, the eighty seconds—top, bottom, two sides. I did up the buttons on my purple coverall and I was back with Tom and he was helping me get into the safety of my green coat. We talked about Astrophysics and Silence. That made sense.

Read *The New Yorker* this afternoon. A horrendous story about Cambodian women going blind for no apparent reason. Their eyes are normal when they are examined, but they can't see. Their story of persecution by the Khmer Rouge is as terrible as the Jewish Holocaust. It is as if they've seen too much and their eyes refuse to look any-

> Without Contraries is no progression. Attraction and Repulsion, Reason and Energy, Love and Hate, are necessary to Human existence.
>
> —*William Blake,*
> *"The Marriage of Heaven and Hell"*

more. It is not coming from childhood trauma. They were happy, simple little girls living with their parents in the rice fields. The author put it down to hysterical blindness, like numbing out when the agony becomes too much.

I think about that. As an anorexic I think I couldn't endure the anguish of life. Too idealistic, yes, but soul killing is not realistic. Even as a child I felt my own soul being killed at school—saw it happening all around me. In Zurich I was told, "Once an anorexic, always an anorexic." Glib! Smart-ass, soul-killing power statement! Soul killing is tragedy. How to avoid it in this culture is a question nobody can answer. Our addictions are our blinders.

On TV, adolescent boys in prison—three had shot their fathers. Because they were minors, they will be out in a few years, and each was swollen with rage—sullen, spiteful, murderous rage. Their souls are forgotten. That's what's tragic. They are like anorexics in that they never thought what would happen to them after they pulled the trigger. They never thought of their own lives destroyed in prison. They all said they just wanted the situation they were in to stop, and they knew no way but death with a gun.

The anorexic wants the horror to stop too. Her way is to starve herself, not that she believes she is dying. Starvation is a metaphor for getting out of an impossible situation—death to the old and maybe hope for the new. But the focus is on stopping the present soul destruction—not being seen, not being heard, no creative space in which to fly. The anorexic takes the rage in and kills herself; the adolescent boys take it out and kill the power-crazy drunken patriarchs who are their fathers or surrogate fathers.

I see it all over. I see myself colluding every time I go for radiation. I collude because I cannot trust my own connection to the positive Great Mother. I have survived in life because I was wary of the destructive forces in my nature that were out to destroy me. That's not true—it was the creative forces that gave up because soul was not recognized. There is the core of the despair. What a trap this is! Negative Mother (withdrawal from life) marries Negative Masculine (the perfect technician), and soul sits on the ceiling saying, "I'll watch, Marion. I may leave." And sweet, holy body, she has no choice but to lie there and take the killing blows. As my doctor says, "We're here to kill."

January 27, 1994

Ross grieves to see me going to radiation, knowing I am going against almost everything within me. It is the conflict I have dealt with all my life. Part of me is tied into the academy, science, perfection; part of me is profoundly connected to the individual soul, nature, imperfection. To go solely the latter route would take great courage. Still, would it be courage when I know my body connection is not trustworthy at the archetypal level? Would it be courage or hubris to fly in the face of science? Is it soul denial? *If* I had the courage, *if* I had the trust in my natural instincts, I would go with the Great Mother and not allow this destruction of my body.

I need to acknowledge that in my December 12 session with Jean I could not get by the *ifs*, and therefore could not surrender to the wisdom of the limbic system, as Jean encouraged me to do. Or, to put it in the imagery of Merton's Buddhist abbot, I dared not leap off the top of the ladder. Fear is still stronger than faith. Forgive me, Sophia.

Tom arrived with another stone from Dory [his wife]. "Hello, Mariannee," he said. I never have to fear we will be late, or that I will have to hurry with my coat. He walks always with his arm near mine or in mine, from the parking lot to the clinic. He sits and reads, and when I return he holds my coat.

I say all this because I took it for granted until Martin took me on Friday. Dear Martin, he kept saying he would get me there on time. We hurtled over the ice in his beautiful van. He put his flashers on and waited for me to run in and get the zap while he sat reading in the loading zone. He is most generous in trying to help me to understand the medical language, and always kind in his own fierce way. He brought sun-ripened Florida grapefruit—twelve of them for healing.

Diego came at 1:15, gave me a bear hug, so glad to see us both, so genuine a smile. Ross and I shocked at his frankness. Diego said everything exactly like it is from a very stark, reduced position. (He and John [sons of Jack and Olga Chambers—both deceased—Jack, a well-known Canadian painter] were here because three of Jack's pictures were bought by the Iveys to give to the London Art Gallery.) John arrived. The sight of him actually took my breath away. Something in his eyes was so like Olga. I felt myself grieving to see her. I saw her in this room four Christmases ago, and all that our friendship was, all that we recognized in each other—all came flooding through in deeper and deeper waves as I saw her playing over his face. To compound this depth, Jack was as present in his face as Olga. That dark, aristocratic aloofness, ruthlessness offset by gentleness with a tragic detachment that never leaves his eyes. Here in the two sons were both Jack and Olga in different degrees at different times.

I think Ross and I were both swept with grief, astonishment, joy, mystery, presences from another world and another time. Time kept going in and out—past, present, future—and from one reality into another. On the walls,

Jack's monumental cat and his double portrait of us listened intently, as if conscious of all Jack had put into them and left them responsible for.

Ross couldn't stop telling them stories of their parents. It was as if we might not be here the next time they come and no one else is alive to tell them what Ross knows of Jack and I know of Olga. We kept our own counsel, but shared all we could. I think we both realized the depth of our love for Jack and Olga, the depth of our love for their children. They were like our own. In remembering our energy when we were all together in this life, something of that energy came back.

Looking at these sensitive young men trying to find their way in a wilderness they don't comprehend, I think of other young people who come to visit. They are equally unwilling to commit to values we took for granted. But what our generation has to answer for! Our greed, our national debt that their generation is going to pay for, if not in money, in life energy. We will look like the patriarchs who sucked their blood out, left them a garbage heap instead of a garden, and poison, literally and symbolically.

Our 5:30 feast was unforgettable. I had no sweets; they don't eat them anyway. I had not been shopping. I had one Brownberry bread loaf and one round Black Diamond cheese. We ate buttered bread and cheese and drank tea and everyone was so hungry and so happy. Long hugs and they went out into the icy night.

January 28, 1994

Put down the check on Sydenham today. No feeling that it is ours. Bad day in every way. Flooding in the streets, ice, rain. Martin took me to the clinic. He is so convinced everything is going to be all right that his unquestioning attitude makes me feel as if he were driving me to buy extra groceries for the weekend. When he was pinching my Latin translations in Grade XII, could we have imagined that we'd be sliding together over the ice in 1994?

January 29, 1994

Jean and I on the phone. Prepared by spending half an hour alone, breathing deep into my belly, concentrating on light energy throughout my skeleton, dropping deeper into my bones and organs and the reptilian section of my brain.

Shamanic Journey: Radiation vs. Inner Healing

The purpose of this journey is to find the voice of the deeper wisdom, the one not connected to the rational voice that keeps throwing up the *ifs*.

I lie in bed and go with it. Jean asks for my images. Ross and lilies, chandelier shining like stars (the one in Lincoln Center). She begins by describing the vault of heaven—the whole of perfection, the great chandelier in the sky, the perfect structure. "Take yourself into that presence," she says. "Go into that perfect vault and find your own highest self—your highest spiritual Marion. See her, look into her face, feel her vibrations."

My whole body begins to vibrate. When the vibrations are well established, she tells me to take that vault to meet my own bodily Marion, who is about sixteen, hair flying in the wind, no illness in her body, no anorexia, no starvation—just huge happy Bubbles energy. I bring the vault to my gut; my own vault is vibrating green. "Healing green, loving green. Let it vibrate green, let it take in the healing vibration." As it vibrates green, I see a woods in spring, bright new greens, snow melting into rivulets, sun dancing off sparkling water. I lie down and allow the cold spring water to flow over me, baptize me. New life coming out of the old—feel my body tingling fresh. Feel the green turning to violet, ultraviolet, feel my vault full of ultraviolet pulsations. Then the vaults come together. These two meet each other in joyous reunion.

Suddenly, my 16-year-old is 22. She cannot trust body. She feels betrayed by body. She does not feel life will cherish her in everlasting arms. Red swirls into orange, swirling fire energy on swirling clouds—sunset before a storm. The energy takes my breath away—swirls into fire. Jean picks up the sunset—day closing, night, preparation for the new day.

I hold, hold, hold. Cherishing arms around me, holding. I am afraid, totally afraid. Gold dust falls from the firmament. I see the light of the chandelier, and I see that light echoed in my kidney—the corona of my healing. I feel the gold going into my kidney and adrenals—I feel fear. CHAOS. Fight or Flight, or paralysis. "Perfect love casteth out fear" (I John 4:18). "Where is that perfect love?"a voice shouts. "You didn't know you had cancer. Don't trust your connection to your body. DO NOT." However much I love the Great Mother, I

Dream, July 23, 1986, Journal Entry

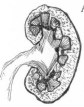 A working kidney appears, surrounded by a mystical light. "Here is the corona of your healing," says a voice.

Dictionary: "corona" 1) a white circle of light seen around a luminous body; 2) the upper portion or crown of a part.

After twelve years of faithfully cherishing my kidney by sending light and love through my palms, perfect love is casting out fear, my snake is connecting to the wheel of life. Edema is no longer armor around my body. Dear God, thank you for the flow.

---

do not trust that I can reach her in the deepest cells in my body. Faith constellated its opposite: fear.

Feel very shaky as that fear registers. Snap into ego. Thank Jean and tell her I will try to rest in those loving arms and talk to her tomorrow. I think she hoped that I could accept the healing from within and stop the radiation. I could not trust from my depths although I believe the cancer is out of my body. The voice instantly comes in: "What if it isn't? And what if the doctor tells you six months from now it has metastasized in your liver and nothing can be done? How foolish would you feel then! If medical science can give you a few years of life, why refuse it?"

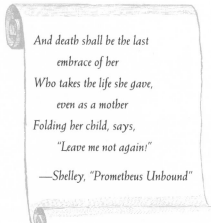

He who binds to himself a joy
Doth the wingéd life destroy
But he who kisses the joy as it flies
Lives in Eternity's sun rise

—William Blake

Yes, I know that sooner or later the Great Mother will take me into her arms in Death, but I do not think this is my time. Maybe the fear is totally unnecessary. So glad not to go to the clinic.

January 30, 1994

Talked to Bruce as he moves to his demanding week in Glasgow. He still has fear of forgetting lines. I would too. I admire his courage—a possible West End production and he hasn't been on the boards for thirty years.

Talked to Margaret, who felt my presence strongly as I wrote to her

And death shall be the last
embrace of her
Who takes the life she gave,
even as a mother
Folding her child, says,
"Leave me not again!"

—Shelley, "Prometheus Unbound"

yesterday. Subtle body connection. She said she tones my name every morning. All this love is so important, because I know I am now able to receive it and my personal issue is love of life versus fear of life.

In this life/death struggle, my darkest corner—infantile abandonment in the womb (therefore lack of connection to Sophia's love in my core)—has reemerged. The conflict that I thought was long since resolved confronts me yet again. The Positive Mother that opens me to oneness and love would carry me into Being in life. The Negative Mother that opens me to rejection and fear would carry me into blank nothingness.

Whether I am being enticed by Christ or the Demon Lover further compounds my angst. Christ says, "I bring you a sword. I come to accompany your incarnated soul into life on Earth. Come with your Beloved." Demon Lover says, "I come to bring you peace. Why suffer this pain? Why remain in this wretched world? Come with your Beloved."

To die: to sleep;
No more; and by a sleep to say we end
The heartache and the thousand natural
*   shocks*
That flesh is heir to. 'Tis a consumma-
tion
Devoutly to be wish'd. To die, to sleep;
To sleep: perchance to dream: ay, there's
*   the rub.*

—Shakespeare, Hamlet

A fierce battle! Positive feminine/masculine at war with negative feminine/masculine: the Royal Marriage versus the Demonic Marriage. Goddess/God is all; Goddess/God is nothing. Life is meaningful; life is meaningless. There's the cosmic paradox.

I read this over and burst into laughter. What a struggle to say so poorly what William said so elegantly four hundred years ago! "To be or not to be" is forever the question. Still, the psychological differentiation does clarify and disperse my fear. I know how deceptive these negative voices can be. If I dialogue with them, I can turn them around.

January 31, 1994

Woke up with the quotation that hung over my childhood bed.

> When the One Great Scorer comes
> to write against your name—
> He marks—not that you won or lost—
> but how you played the game.
>
> —Grantland Rice

That gives me pause. I absorbed that more deeply than I realized. I never thought of the Scorer as a judge tallying up failures against me. No! He simply tallied points on both sides. How I played the game was what made me who I am. Playing cancer is no different. Don't fall into either/or thinking, Marion. Stay with the feminine both/and.

February 1, 1994

Joanne is driving me to the clinic this week. We laugh as we laughed for twenty years together on the South Staff. She is faithful as the Rock of Gibraltar.

In my dream she and I arrive at the customs office as we cross into Detroit. Dark. No light anywhere. I am driving. Suddenly an evil presence, totally invisible, speaks through my open window: "Give me everything you've got." Joanne, sitting beside me, says, "Give him the four hundred dollars you've got in your bra and step on the accelerator." I do, and we shoot out of his reach with our purses under our seats intact.

That's Joanne—fast, intelligent decisions, fearless and sensible against impossible odds. She walks on the earth; I tend to fly. That makes for great laughs because our humor comes out of her trying to fly and my trying to stay flat on the ground.

As we cross the border into unknown territory, we are confronted by dire evil, evil so dire it is not even personified. It demands everything. My healthy shadow, Joanne (who sensibly carries four hundred dollars in her bra whenever she travels), recognizes there is no point in attempting to fight this presence. Redirect its energy by giving it the full feminine four and get out with our identity and our jewels intact. She recognizes the difference between collective evil, which is too immense for one person to battle, and personal evil, which needs to be dealt with. That discrimination and decisiveness I need in establishing new priorities during this time of healing. It is equally important to waste no time dithering in the face of overwhelming darkness.

Glowing spring garden from Johanne and Shirley—daffodils, hyacinths, red tulips singing in every direction. I let them stand and fall as they wish.

February 4, 1994

Disoriented as I went to the clinic. As I walked across the parking lot, my child's voice started in me. "I don't like this, Marion. We've had too much radiation. You can walk me right up to Sarah and you can sign in, but I'm not going

to go through the big doors." I kept walking right up to
Sarah. Again the voice: "I told you, Marion, I'm not going
in." I could almost feel this child dragging on my coat.

"I seem to have a problem here," I said to Sarah. "I think
I'll just sit down for a minute."

"Are you not well?" she asked.

"Tell her we're not going in for radiation today." The
child is almost shouting.

"I don't think I'm able to do the radiation today," I said.

"Oh, that's all right," Sarah said. "The doctor was considering canceling your sessions until next Tuesday."

Little One was turning somersaults and laughing with
glee.

Home with Joanne, laughing about our trip to Egypt
with the South students. The day we went to the pyramids
most of them had diarrhea. Nothing to do but stop the bus
every five minutes. No pride in the ditch and sweet compassion in the bus.

The body does not lie.

February 10, 1994

Aidan's first birthday. Could I ever forget the entry of
that tiny beauty into this world? There in their own home,
Richard and I, with the midwives, accompanied Marion
through her travail, the bone-chilling screams, the final ecstasy of agony and triumph—and for me, concentration on
her rather than on the new life relentlessly pushing through
the pain. Then the little head crowned, and waited, and
then fast appeared, one arm and then another as we caught
his swinging little body with its bluish skin.

Yes, dear Aidan. How exquisite! How innocent! How
you have the right—like every child born—to a life in har-

> *Our birth is but a sleep and a*
>> *forgetting:*
>>> *The Soul that rises with us, our*
>>>> *life's Star,*
> *Hath had elsewhere its setting,*
>> *And cometh from afar:*
> *Not in entire forgetfulness,*
> *And not in utter nakedness,*
> *But trailing clouds of glory do we come*
>> *From God, who is our home:*
> *Heaven lies about us in our infancy!*
> *Shades of the prison house begin to close*
>> *Upon the growing Boy.*
>
>> *—William Wordsworth,*
>> *"Ode: Intimations of Immortality"*

mony with nature: forest, frost, winter branches, rain, river, rock—the flesh and bone of Earth.

How you should have the right to wander in the woods in perfect freedom, perfect communion, to walk down the street in safety, to enjoy strangers, to stretch your arms and legs and head to the fullness of your whole Being. No constrictions, no fear.

But it is not so, dear little boy. I think of you. I think of the news. I wonder what you will see in your lifetime—you with your blue eyes, so trusting, so sensitive, and your blond hair and fair skin, so asking to be caressed.

Dear little fellow, bang your pots and pans and your Mickey Mouse telephone. Enjoy freedom in your soul. "Shades of the prison house" will come soon enough.

Paul phoned. I feel his deep concern. I also feel his incapacity to deal with my having *cancer.* That word undermines the children—childhood years of anguish for their mother and later anguish for their father. Shelley's reaction to my cancer was to go to the woods, find a small limb of birch, speak to it, saw it off, carve it with specific healing runes, and stain it with red ocher. This finely wrought bindrune she brought to me with Lauren's carved candlestick. This done, she fled to Florida. Too close to the bone! Still, whatever else, I shall be eternally thankful to Shelley for her calls to California that brought us home. Had Fraser died with no ritual journey, no farewell, I would have had to deal with guilt as well as grief.

Sang with Marion Rose on the phone. Heard her afterward, as I spoke with Paul, "Rock, rock, rocking," belting out our song in her rocker.

February 12, 1994

Nancy phoned to encourage me to eat sprouted seeds (essential for enzymes) and sea vegetables. So many people are helping me all in their own way. Ann sends me a card with an archetypal message every two weeks. As I become weaker, Love keeps me in life.

Lena, dear Lena, was here all day. After twenty years of coming twice a month, she knows exactly what is necessary to clean the house. I was extremely tired, so just did the flowers before she came—roses in champagne glasses in the bathrooms. How I love an alive bathroom! And an alive closet! Created a total mess getting Ross's closet into operation as closet again. Spent yesterday throwing things out or sending them to the cleaners or to Goodwill. Discriminating all the way. That done, fell asleep.

I know in my cells that prayer permeates a sick body, makes it shimmer as the new life comes in, making the cells remember how to respond to the harmonic whole. Music is like prayer—a

The physical substance evolves through each individual formation, and one day, it will be capable of bridging the gap between the physical life as we know it and the supramental life that will manifest.

—Mother, quoted in Satprem,
The Mind of the Cells

mystical bridge between heaven and earth. I guess all art, all genuine religions are born of the subtle body that is the connector between divine and human.

"Thinning the membrane calls us to a memory of something we've never consciously known. We know it by its absence. This is the presence that absence leaves." I don't know where that is from, but I do know that as this radiation continues, we are "thinning the membrane" and I am becoming increasingly aware of the reality on the other side that I have always known by its absence.

February 13, 1994

Quiet Sunday.

My dear friends are realizing I'm becoming more exhausted by the radiation. They don't phone on Sunday as they did before.

Ross and I watched the opening of the Olympic Games in Lillehammer, Norway, last night. Thrilling to see all those radiant young faces marching together, here to give their all through the discipline that brings out the very best that is in them—competing, living in the same village. Surely this in an antidote for war. It brings out nationalism and competitive spirit in the best possible way. Norwegian flags are red above the crowd.

Dark underbelly to all of this. Sarajevo, where the Games were held in '84, is under threat. The UN and NATO have ordered the Serbs to have their big guns off the surrounding hills by midnight, February 20. All the love that is being manifested in these Games was once mani-

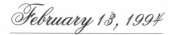

The answer, my friend, is writ in the wind,

The answer is writ in the wind.

fested in Sarajevo. The cameras pan across the great stadium—bombed out, an empty shell. Suddenly I see Torvill and Dean glide out onto the ice like two bluebirds. Freedom in motion. As the pulse of *Bolero* intensifies and climaxes, I and tens of thousands of others around the world weep in the presence/absence of the oneness of two shining flames. Ten/ten across the board. Ice dancing is forever changed. Ten years ago, all that glory gleamed in the center of what is now a cemetery for the dead killed in a ferocious attack. What sense does it make?

Cheered the skier leaping into full flight to light the Olympic flame. Enchanted when the vast layer of white snow suddenly shimmered with movement. Gradually, so gradually, the trolls pushed their way through, usually backside first. So Norwegian, so Viking, so mischievous, so droll! I love the way these golden-haired, blue-eyed angels always hold on to the underbelly of their gold. The trolls moved into dancing with the angel children in their native costumes. Felt Sonja's [deceased sister-in-law's] Norwegian blood pulsing!

I love it! I love it! Too exhausted to do anything right now, so feel guiltless as I spend hours focused on these concentrated young faces, so vital and happy. And all these smiling Norwegians, so full of fresh cows' milk and healthy bread and cheese—their effort and caring give new hope for the world. The great egg that slowly descended through

Images provide messages that are understood by the immune system. They link conscious thoughts with the white blood cells in such a way that the appropriate combinations and numbers come rushing forth to perform in ways that not even the most knowledgeable immunologist could command.

—*Jeanne Achterberg,*
Imagery in Healing

the darkness of the northern snows gradually lit up from the inside, gradually opened, and released a white dove. Sublime as the snowflakes fell! Then several thousand helium balloons in the shape of doves ascended. PEACE. Dear God, I hope so.

Strange, Ross and I both said we would really like some chocolate (we never mention chocolate from one year's end to another anymore). Here we are on Valentine's Eve, yearning for that verboten chocolate.

February 14, 1994

Lots of Victorian valentines. Feel so upheld by the everlasting arms of love—human and divine—part of each other, no ultimate separation. So necessary to open to this love. Returning to the clinic today. Sometimes, as I go, I feel this will never be over. I will always be afraid of the cancer, always unable to allow myself coffee, raw vegetables, and raw fruit. I have to remember this is only for three more weeks, this radiation, this tiredness, this darkness of winter. I can understand the moment when the effort to eat exactly, take the exact pills, make the right decisions for health and life becomes too much. But I dare not allow myself to think that way. Nor do I dare to allow myself to think about Mary [deceased friend] and the anguish I now understand even more—the anguish of the aloneness of death.

Bruce's exquisite valentine also arrived. I phoned Bill Posno [florist] two weeks ago and told him I knew flowers would probably be arriving. "Please, no arranged bouquets," I said. I can't bear to see flowers cut and twisted on wires and jammed in a vase so not one of them has a chance to show off its own glory and no way to collect its own strength from its own stem. No, I like to see them tall and free. I like to arrange them in different vases as they fade so their aging patina matches the patina of the vase. Red roses in their aging love pewter. There's where I can see myself and honor my aging. Bill heard me. Bruce's long-stemmed daisies, lilies, carnations, freesia arrived with a box of four big Victorian chocolates. "The best chocolate in the world," the box said.

Our verboten chocolate! We instantly had a taste. Oh glory be! Just like the box said! I took one to David [nephew], who is driving me this week in his vehicle. Dear soul, he was out in the courtyard dusting the snow off his windows and trying to get some of the clutter from the cab into the back of the truck. We talked about his dreams. He seems free and glad to talk. Noreen [his friend] will take me twice this week.

Chocolate is a bean; therefore, chocolate is a vegetable. So there!

Bruce opened in Aberdeen today. Full of memories of our journey to Scotland with Mother and Father. He loves touring in those great old theaters.

I am giving up my office at 223 St. Clair. The time is more than ripe. I shall miss Toronto.

Dear Sophia, please keep your shield over my belly and over my heart. Yes, over my eyes. I feel somewhat blind after the treatment. Please protect my skin. Please protect my bowels from being burned. Please protect me from permanent damage through human error. Fill me with ultraviolet light. Let me take on as much of the higher energies as possible without damage to my body. Thank you. Thank you for your love that forever upholds me. Thank you for the special love that came to me this day. Thank you for fifteen years in Toronto.

February 15, 1994

Mary took me today. I do look forward to my drivers.
By the time we get to where we're going, I've forgotten
we're going to the gas chamber. "Business first," Mary said.
(Oh, yes. I gave her one of the big chocolates to take on
her trip to California where I might have been and whence
I returned when Fraser was moving into Death. She said too
bad I didn't have one for Ann, who is going too and has a
passion for chocolate. She said they'd divide it as a communion.)

So business first: we talked about Abraxas [intensive
workshop] and whether it would be possible. I agreed to
try it, to try to find a new way. Yes! I felt I might get into
the swing again. She told me a friend of hers told her that
Marion is known at the clinic as the patient who asks all the
impossible questions. I wish I'd known a few more before I
got into this. Anyway, felt so good with Mary driving
through the heavy snow, she all wrapped in her gray down
coat, and I in my green Victorian. Good talking business
too.

Then I went in for my treatment. Came out. Twenty
seconds on each side, eighty seconds altogether.

Mary stared at me. "You've been zapped," she said.
"Your energy is completely different. You look as if you
can't walk. Shall I bring the car to the door on the lower
level?"

"No," I said. "I need to try."

But I knew I couldn't climb the stairs, so we took the elevator to the wrong floor. One person went to the clinic;
another was brought home. I saw some terrible cases
today—one man with half his face eaten off, another with
huge lumps eating his arm (a young, handsome man). Oh
dear, oh dear, it made me glad I was doing radiation, al-

though what ultimate harm it may be doing I don't know. As my doctor says, "We're here to destroy. Yes, twenty years from now—fifteen maybe—there may be reactions in your body. It won't matter then." Got the message, Marion?

When I come in, Ross looks at me to see how dizzy I am. "You're going to have a sleep," he says. I do, sometimes for the whole afternoon. I make supper and go to bed again. Can work only between 5:00 A.M. and 8:00 A.M. and that not too clearly. Went for a half-hour walk today, but it was too much.

February 16, 1994

David drove me again in a storm. I decided to wait to see Dr. Thomas. He hasn't come to see me since our encounter over the "something in the liver," so I decided to stay today until he came for our interview. This is the man whom I am to meet every six months for five years.

After my treatment, I sat and read "A Patient's Guide to Radiation Therapy." Then I heard him laughing with a nurse in the hall. He walked in.

"I waited," I said, "because I think there should be some relationship between doctor and patient. We are to meet over the next few years. Healing is a two-way thing."

"Yes, I'll be seeing you every six months," he said.

"*You* will?" I asked.

He got the implication. "Yes, I will," he said. He ignored my thoughts about the healer/patient relationship.

"I am very worried about my forty-eight-hour intensive," I said, "because I cannot lie still for that long and I am already so burned. I don't know if I can take any more without permanent damage."

"We will take care of your being still," he said. "If you move and the nodes move, this could cause very serious, permanent damage. You'll be still. Then I won't see you for another six months."

"I hope that's true," I said.

A PATIENT'S GUIDE TO RADIATION THERAPY

Brachytherapy for cancer of the cervix and/or uterus

What is brachytherapy?

Brachytherapy is a form of radiation treatment in which special applicators deliver radiation as close to a tumor as possible.

Is hospitalization necessary?

Yes because a patient undergoing brachytherapy requires general anesthetic, because the treatment is conducted in a specially equipped room and because it can last up to forty-eight hours. Insurance covers a private room for brachytherapy and the hospital stay can vary, sometimes lasting up to five days.

What happens during the treatment?

While the patient is under general anesthesia, the special applicators are inserted into the vagina and/or uterus. After the procedure is over and the patient is alert, she is taken back to her room. There the applicators are hooked up to long tubes that are connected to a machine which delivers the radioactive material to the applicators. The doctor determines the length of therapy time, which varies from patient to patient. Sometimes radioactive materials are put directly into the vagina and/or uterus.

What should patients bring to the hospital?

A patient should bring any medications she is taking but should leave all valuables behind. To while away the time, a patient should bring reading materials, small handicrafts, crossword puzzles, portable cassette players and the like. Televisions and phones can be rented.

At least we're honest with each other. Always the double entendre. We'll both rejoice if we don't see each other for six months because I'll be free of cancer and we don't need to see each other. In these moments of dread, I am mesmerized by his total otherness as I suspect he is by mine.

"I won't be bringing paint by numbers," I said.

"As you wish," he said, and left.

That comment comes out of meeting with the nurse. She gives me a brochure. She tells me radiation won't harm a Walkman or tapes. I may bring a paint-by-numbers kit.

Is this not primitive? Is it not like being buried alive in an initiation ceremony? And on the third day I rise again, resurrected, if I survive the ordeal. My Walkman will be safe!

Come to think of it, this is not so primitive. This is my Easter weekend, although Easter is a month away. I won't take anything but some tapes and one book. I wish I had my own little New Testament here. It's on my altar in Toronto. India again! There I had my passport to read aloud, my Shakespeare sonnets, my New Testament.

When I returned to the waiting room, David was concentrating on the fish. Together we dropped into their silent world. His gentle strength supported me as we rumbled back to Windermere. We talked about my desk that Father created for me "out of the first organ to come to Huron County from Scotland." I told him how proud his grandfather had been that his family loved music enough to bring that organ from Scotland. It must have come at huge expense—the cost of the organ, plus the shipping—to a family that had virtually nothing but a bee apiary and trees to cut down for house and barn. He couldn't bear to see the organ disposed of, so he made it into a desk. I remember him in Norwich, working so patiently, sanding, rubbing with his big hands and a rag, resanding, rubbing, resanding, rubbing, down to an exquisite finish. What a patient, cherishing man he was! How much he accomplished, although nothing ever hurried him!

As I told David the story, I realized that desk has been a bulwark at the center of my life. I can't bear to see it disposed of. Ross has never liked it much, but now that I've emptied out all the drawers, he suddenly sees how valuable it has been throughout our 35 years of marriage in keeping us organized. Each drawer is the right size for special things—passports, income tax receipts, keys, special videos, special photos, tapes, old magazines—Charles and Diana's engagement, Charles and Diana's wedding, Churchill's funeral—*Life* magazines marking the great occasions. Well, there isn't room for the desk in the new house, so the dispersal begins now. No place to store anything either, so we have to clear now. Marion says she really wants that desk, so David will come tomorrow with his truck to take it to her in Toronto.

What a time of clearing to essence! This emptying feels like a purge. My body, my soul, my spirit are emptying. I can even feel some excitement about entering darkness, allowing darkness to penetrate my depths.

> When the temple is cleared of every hindrance, . . . of strangers and their properties, its appearance is beautiful and it shines so clear and pure . . . that no one but the uncreated God can be reflected in it.
>
> —*Meister Eckhart*

February 17, 1994

A nun I do not know sent me my own prayer today—something she had read in one of my books: "Let me burn in the fire—further cleansing, finer tuning." Be careful what you pray for, Marion. Your prayer may be answered.

Thinking more about Cherry's letter today. In it she said: "I can empathize with your sense of betrayal, your rage at your body for betraying you—your body with which you have had such an ambiguous relationship all your life. Now, after you've worked so hard to create a loving relationship with it, it has broken down in cancer. No wonder you would be raging!" That's her projection. I let my rage go over twenty years ago in India when I consciously chose to stay in my body rather than forsake her. Raging would be sheer histrionics now.

Still, I'm glad Cherry wrote; she made me realize I have no sense of rage against my body, no sense of its having betrayed me. In fact, the opposite is true. I believe it is my best friend. I knew something irrevocable had happened when I fell on the rock. That fall saved me from the ravages of advanced cancer. I think God spoke directly to me through that fall. Instantly, I knew the fall was from within. I had to "let go and let God." To fall into the arms of the living God is an awesome fall. Looking back, I see all the signposts pointing to a new level of surrender. No, I feel no rage toward my body. My soul dwells in my body; however tenuous their relationship, they are my path to God and Sophia, circuitous as that path may be.

In summary, here was the initiation route, once the constellation began to move from unconscious into consciousness:

> The mystery of the Virgin Mother lies in her fiat, her acceptance of life's experiences. . . . It is this experience that links Inanna, Kore, Mary and Sophia who descend into life and become of one nature with it.
>
> —*Caitlín Matthews,*
> Sophia: Goddess of Wisdom

Separation	1) fall (separation from the collective group)
Entering sacred space	2) resting in God's grace on the island (the beginning of limbo—liminal space betwixt and between worlds)
	3) attempt to return to the collective, thwarted by severe pain (recognition of meridian connection between knees and womb)
	4) yearning to go to England—take acupuncture almost daily in Toronto for three weeks in order to be able to walk
	5) appearance of a few drops of blood—initiation into Cronedom?
	6) return home to London, Ont., to see Dr. Cohen, whom I recently found—she will set up appointment with gynecologist while I am away
Thanksgiving	7) to London, England—work out every morning on Bruce's stationary bike—walk or ride in wheelchair. Love London as if I'll never see it again. Ross and I do workshop on the complementary union of opposites—spirit and matter. Opens new dimension in our marriage
	8) return to Canada—see Dr. Fellows next day
In sacred space	9) cancer
Sacrifice and Scarification Body mutation	10) womb sacrificed—no pain in legs or back, legs no longer hanging on my body like sacks of potatoes, thank legs for early cancer diagnosis—new energy pouring through knees into tips of toes—energy pouring into new standpoint
Seclusion chamber	11) radiation—further body mutation—holding tension of opposites (losing past; questioning future) (bodysoul/spirit shift)—metamorphosis in process, choosing new wholeness in attempting to hold spiritual womb always receptive to creative spirit

12) just ahead—who knows? Is there any return to the collective?

I'm silent in the face of God's mysterious workings through events and symptoms. My body has always been the instrument through which I have been forced to come to consciousness (heatstroke, eating addiction, car accident, kidneys, knees, cancer).

Body has been the instrument of initiation that made clear what my sacrifice must be, where the new threshold stood open, how the new vision might manifest. Its agony forced me onto a new path, where I did not want to go. Or rather, I could scarcely go because I was chained by a complex to a present which had become a past. I yearned for the New Day but felt powerless to get out of what I was in *graciously.* Always through illness God picked me up, dropped me on the new road, and said, "Walk!"

Dear Sophia, help me to walk on the ground. I love my dear body—"a poor thing, but mine own." Prospero probably said that about Caliban.

I shouldn't say that. It is not beautiful by collective standards. But it is noble, intelligent, and fiercely intuitive, with limitless sense of fun. It behaves like Gyronne [deceased Cairn]. He would jump into the Volvo with greatest glee, but if he realized we were on our way to the vet, he would nuzzle his way in behind me, his little body shaking from ears to tail. However closely I held him, telling him it was for his own good, he shook and could not trust me. He seemed so alone, so tiny a mite trying to hold on to his bit of life in my arms. My body acts exactly the same way. Thursday I stepped up confidently to the receptionist. She asked me to sign something; I saw the red lights flashing on the No Entry room; my hand was shaking so much I couldn't write. Sheer terror in the presence of high-tech machinery. The Unknown God!

Terrific conflict every time I go. I can't endure hurting my dear animal. One-sixteenth of a mistake and I could be on a colostomy bag for the rest of my life! My doctor warned me of that. I pray to Sophia before I go in and all the time I'm there. Then I dance out, sometimes into a wall, but dizzy or not dizzy, thankful to her.

I always ask my body's forgiveness for taking her to radiation. I don't know. . . . I think of Chan [Mother's Siamese bluepoint]. Will I ever forget the look of forgiveness that breathed from his blue eyes into my mother's blue eyes as I drove them to the vet when he was too sick to live? He didn't squirm or fight. He lay in her arms, never once taking his eyes from hers—utter love, although he knew she was taking him to his death. That cat had such uncanny intuition I know he understood.

When we got there, Mother bravely carried him in; I surreptitiously carried his box. I heard her tell the vet she couldn't do it yet. "When you are ready, Mrs. Boa," the vet said. She carried Chan to a nearby field to talk to him. I could see them communing with each other in total love. It was too sacred to watch—this parting with her soul animal. Then she brought him in, gave him to the vet, and within five minutes, his box containing his little cat body was handed to her.

The Lord gave, and the Lord hath taken away; blessed be the name of the Lord.

—*Job* 1:21

Through staying with her feminine timing and honoring their love for each other, Mother came home forgiven. I will defend these same values, whatever happens. I will not be ravaged by guilt. Transition begins in forgiveness.

Something very important is trying to get through to me as I write this. My body is letting go, remembering my love for little Gyronne. Muscles are relaxing; energy is flowing, warm, deep. The image is transforming the energy in my body, the same image that saved my life when I was dying in the Ashoka in India. In that near-death experience, from my position on the ceiling, I suddenly found myself looking into the innocent eyes of my dog looking out of my own rejected body on the floor. Instantly I loved her as I loved him. She IS my body. I forgave her all her sins (sins no more), came off the ceiling, and chose embodiment.

Now I am asking her to forgive me. In remembering those two cherishing animals, I am living forgiveness in my body. She is flowing with love for me because she is not rejected. We are whole.

Is this what forgiveness is? Forgiveness initiated these two transitions: I forgave my body in India; she is forgiving me now. I think to forgive is to transform what we would otherwise reject. The acceptance here is in the connection between the eyes: Presence leads to Resonance leads to Acceptance leads to Love. By Love I mean Reality—that which is True. I am understanding "Beauty is Truth, Truth Beauty" as I never experienced it in my cells before. The resonance is the knowing.

Yes, I understand something else. I need to change my visualization. Instead of pouring red-hot spirit energy into my already radiated pelvis, I need to visualize cool, flowing

I saw it [my body] lying there helpless, still, and then I saw it take in a breath. "Poor dummy," I thought. "Don't you know you're dead?" . . . Suddenly I remembered my little Cairn terrier. . . . I wouldn't treat a dog the way I'm treating my own body.

—Marion Woodman,
The Pregnant Virgin

water or moonlight. "Yes," she says, "oh, yes. Thank you for hearing." I feel the unity of physical body and spirit in subtle body in love.

7:00 P.M.

Spent two days on the phone talking to different companies about water—deionized, distilled, filtered. So difficult to find the information necessary to make a decision. Have decided to put twelve hundred dollars into Aquathin and build it into the kitchen at Sydenham. If I'm to drink two quarts of water a day in order to live, I'm not going to drink polluted or chlorinated water. Besides, the Aquathin feels like velvet slipping down my throat.

Meeting people is becoming increasingly difficult. I can't "prepare a face to meet" a face. I need to fall into my own nothingness to rest. A pregnant emptiness. A forever aloneness. That's why airports are so important in my dreams. In their vast, noisy domain, everyone has left somewhere and not arrived anywhere. I can be totally present in that space between—here is only the present I create for myself in reading or writing or conversation. Here is no elsewhere to which I long to escape. Like the ocean voyages I once loved, here is untrammeled elsewhere, free of the past, free of the future. NOW.

I do not fear aloneness. I do not fear the lead chamber. Essentially we are all always alone. Listened to Callas singing Norma. The emptiness/fullness of a cathedral dome opened. Her aloneness—her forever aloneness is her power. However much she tried to belong—driving herself to thinness, connecting to a man—the uniqueness of her voice is the tragic aloneness that permeates every aria. She opens to another dimension of fullness. Keats's "full-throated ease." Destiny—to live one's destiny with graciousness.

February 18, 1994

Ross asked me why I am pasting all these old pictures in this book. "They're all I can keep of the hundreds," I say. I just realized the ones I've chosen are all rite of passage pictures—essence pictures, no persona. I need to know that person that emerged from each initiation. I need to look her in the eyes now and see her as she has matured.

"But," says Ross, "no one will ever see them. You say all your journals are in your lawyer's office ready to go up in flames if anything happens to you. And this one will be no different."

"They are for myself," I say. "I need to do the work on myself for myself in order to get through the initiation. Clearing these old albums brings their story inside, instead of leaving it in projection in the photograph. I'm integrating pieces of my lifetime, providing a loving mirror for who I AM at each threshold."

So back to my pictures. The smiling one was taken in the middle of the night in our kitchen at 380. Wayne [friend] and I, having laughed our way around Covent Garden [London, Ont.] buying peaches, three bushels of them, were preparing peaches for the freezer. Luscious fruit, so sensuous! *Peach*. Even the word opens into a blossom on the lips, a sensuous blossom ready to be plucked in full femininity. He was on his way to Harvard the next day, and we were having a joyous and deadly serious night putting peaches in boiling water, slipping off the skins, and putting them in plastic bags for the freezer. That's what we were doing as we talked of his going and my staying.

Wayne holds as much agony as I do. He loves beauty as I do. He is as detached as I am because he has to be to survive. He is one side of Ross in my life, with all his aesthetic sense, his love of drama, his profound surrender to dance. But I am not married to Wayne, and therefore there is nothing to lose with him even if we both went over the edge of a cliff in our dancing. So we can live our cherishing of each other, experience the delight of each other's rebellion against the collective, be surprised by what comes spluttering out of our mouths, know the agony but not focus on it, or focus on it and move it into the absurd and laugh until we cry—two lone creatures, way, way out.

Wayne was there to meet me when I arrived in Boston from India, striding toward him in my Jaeger coat—free, free, free, "nothing left to lose." We went to his apartment where regal lilies blessed the table and the champagne and fruits. Whatever would I have done without the few precious playmates I found on the way—playmates as far-out and as broken as I was. But not broken at all in the aloneness that was my strength, as their aloneness was theirs.

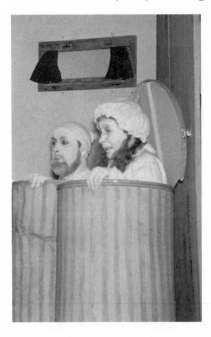

NAGG: Yesterday you scratched me there.
NELL: (elegiac): Ah, yesterday!

—*Samuel Beckett*, Endgame.

Beckett is the world Wayne and I share. It is also the world Ross and I share when we are not too seriously involved in our marriage. Ross and I love the absurd, and his black humor is the funniest I know, but we have to come back to the reality that we are married. We do live in a world where bills have to be paid, dishes done, and suicide is not an acceptable escape. So I can play out with Wayne what eventually would become fatal with Ross (though we have mellowed in our later years). Beckett! How often now Ross explodes in frustration with Nagg's line "I had it yesterday." And I respond with Nell's rhapsodic "Ah, yesterday." There we are—Ross and I in the garbage cans we climbed into three different years to play our Beckett roles. Well, we aren't onstage now. We simply are.

Then the other two pictures. The passport picture was taken after the car accident that nearly killed us both. Again, the sense of fatality! I played with the electric windows on our way to the party, thank God, and knew how to work them when it came time to decide whether we were in the river or on land when we had to climb out of the upside-down Cadillac. As he spoke in the old Colonel Talbot house, Ross knew there was going to be trouble at the bridge that night. We actually did cross the bridge safely with our drunk driver. Then he decided to go back to get the forgotten money box and crashed into the side of the bridge driving like a banshee. The car hit the bridge exactly where I was sitting. There's my head put back together by that great surgeon who cut through my scalp and pulled the bones back into place.

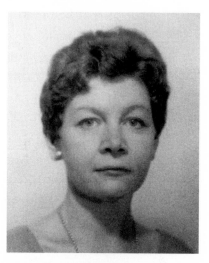

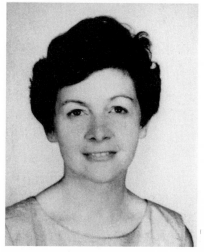

Ross looks at the picture and says, "That never was you." But I think it was. The accident was in May '68. I already had my ticket for around the world. By the middle of July I was determined to go, because I could not stay in London, neither accept nor escape its conventional values. I could not stay to be haunted by what once I was that now, like a ghost, continually questioned and undermined what I was trying to become. I was hidden, even from myself. There I am unable to smile, the nerves on the left side of my face paralyzed. That steady, strong gaze knows I have to go whatever the outcome. Fear was beside the point. Of course I was terrified, but I had to leave the known that was destroying me with its comforts and plush hypocrisy. My Gypsy had to dance.

That aloneness turns into the aloneness of India—the other picture—the visa picture I had to get in order to go to Teheran. An Indian photographer took it. It is the face that came out of the initiation in the Ashoka Hotel. Gone is the "I will be perfect. I will be a scholar, I will be beautiful. I will make my body what I want it to be. I will, I will, I will." Every line of my body speaks of the sacrifice of that driving willpower that had been destroying me. Because I had conquered the fear of Death, I was no longer constellating Death in the street. I had *surrendered* my ego desires to Sophia's love. "Thy will be done."

February 19, 1994

"So what am I doing spending so much time with these pictures?" I ask myself. Practically speaking, I am clearing out what is of no value to anyone after I'm dead, letting irrelevant matter go. Lightening up, *simplifying* in order to concentrate on essentials.

At the same time, I am honoring life by trying to bring more consciousness into my own journey. I am seeing the archetypal dimensions that have forced me toward wholeness against my will. I am seeing the progression of spirals through which I have moved upward and downward, higher into spirit, deeper into grounding. What a paradox is there: flying higher into heaven, at the same time being forced to work deeper into the hell of my addiction, the hell of my own unconscious body. Just when I thought I was once again in balance, I would find myself face to face with another threshold guarded by the angels and demons of the unconscious. To survive, I had to leap. And leap I did—right out of the jaws of the archetypal demonic parents and into the arms of unknowing. Each leap brought me closer to my own soul, my own bone, and my inner royal parents. This cancer is another threshold leading to a new round of the spiral. What an incredible map I seem to have followed! I am silenced by its intricacies.

Repressed energy returns to haunt us in symbol and symptom.

—MW

Looking carefully at these pictures, I can see that when body is vacated by spirit, Presence is absent. I remember the story of Marilyn Monroe walking down the street with a friend. No one noticed her. The friend was astonished and asked Marilyn if she was aware of this. "Do you want to see them look at me?" she asked. Then she concentrated, began to radiate energy, and people suddenly began to crowd around her. Stars are concentrated enough to focus their own light. Concentration is related to simplifying. In this moment, this and this only. Presence. Here. Now.

This healing is about spiritual energy penetrating matter, two different frequencies of energy. Without my visualizations, I could become a lethargic crocodile, and that old Mother would quickly pull me into everlasting mud. Visualization and prayer open my body to the energy of spirit—

feminine opening to masculine. When my spirit becomes too intense for my body (when I am in deep mourning or when I am midwifing someone through death), my body is far more vulnerable than I recognize. That can be also true when I read poetry, listen to music, concentrate on art. Spirit can move into another dimension and leave body behind. My body is outraged—no, it is enraged. That's where real trouble starts. Our culture is likewise plagued with this split. In most people it remains unconscious. Then they are shocked when their autoimmune systems turn against them or they wonder why they are victims of their addictions. A forsaken body carries a suicidal drive.

February 20, 1994

Olav, the Norwegian hero, sped to victory today. Talk about a star concentrating on his own light! Olav is a great Viking prince—golden hair, blue eyes, burning fire waiting for the gun to go off so he can start his indomitable rhythm toward his goal. Terrific! That's the only kind of spirit to have if you want to be a winner. You have to be responsible to your own vision. If you make yourself dependent on others, you are setting yourself up for betrayal. But then I think of Christ. He was betrayed by almost all, but that's when His reality shone brightest. That must be left in God's hands.

Olav was glorious. Glide after glide, his big, powerful legs sped to their goal, as if his inner harmony were in tune with some greater harmony. Falling for him was unthinkable. He knew. He didn't once think of failure. He won.

Torvill and Dean came third in the technical. All kinds of judging politics! For me, they transcend skating, soul in movement. But I realized something. Maybe they have become too perfect, too locked in their own perfection, that terrifying point where perfect beauty cannot open itself to spontaneity and love. The Russian pair, Gordeeva and Grinkov, love each other and their love is in every gesture, every radiant look. How I envy people who can express their love for each other in that way—through the discipline of the work they both love. If that happens to be through the body—oh, the ecstasy!

The cameramen are exquisite in portraying the subtle body relationship of G and G. They are working in a different dimension—the reality of the shifting relationship that moves their skates. Maybe that is what Elvis is talking about when he "skates from the heart," and the judges haven't seen it yet. Kurt Browning is finding it. And little Oksana Baiul "waits for her skates to tell her to start." Maybe this is waiting for spirit to enter matter in order that God's timing may be incarnated. I really feel the dense physical is balanced by the high etheric in these games. Seeing these radiant young people is the best medicine I could possibly have.

February 21, 1994

Went shopping at Loblaws, carried bags. Gut is red-hot bubbling, growling—Blake's Bowlahoola [god of digestion] telling me he doesn't like bags at all. Going to stay on vegetable mush and custards.

These are days of "warm up, melt down." I hope my burnt body doesn't go through meltdown after radiation.

I'm realizing that healing won't be like it was after the operation—cut out the tumor and then depend on the wisdom
of the cells for healing. No, radiation weakens the body,
leaves scars, leaves residue. I'll try to work with the healing
in a different way.

Sylvia and Pam are driving me this last week. Very at-
tentive, very caring.

February 22, 1994

Willows covered with hoarfrost on the river.

The nurse at the clinic this morning said she would take
care of me.

"No," I said, "I'll wait until my doctor comes."

So he came. Soul did not meet soul.

"Will you bring your paint by numbers?" he asked as he
came in.

"You know I don't paint by numbers," I said. "My cells
sing when they know they can paint anything any way."

"You might get too excited," he said. "No paints."

A first robin was cheer-upping on the lawn outside.

"Don't you think I would cheer up at the thought of
seeing you every six months if we had some understanding? Wouldn't you cheer up at the thought of seeing me?
Alive?"

"Not at all," he said. "I don't understand that. Don't understand anything about stress causing cancer either. If stress
caused cancer, we'd all be dead. We're all stressed out."

He made a dramatic stressed-out gesture that made me
laugh.

"I may not do the lead vault," I said. "If my dreams tell
me not to, I'll phone to say I'm not coming."

"It's up to you," he said. "We cut out the treatment for some years and the results were not good. Do as you please."

I have to say I quite like the man. Blunt and harsh as he can be, he is honest.

I saw the little boy whose mother brings him to the clinic every day in a wagon. He's getting smaller and weaker, and more angelic every day. He smiles at me and I smile at him, and I can hardly hold my tears. I'm sure my doctor has to be brutal with his own feelings in order to survive at all.

February 23, 1994

Fragrant spring air! Snowdrops whispering together in the garden. Shocked to realize how fearful my feet are of stepping on the ground and terrified of crossing the street. I stand looking at the green light and say, "Now it's OK, Sweethearts. You've received a hard blow, but nothing is going to hurt you here." I try to breathe into them to hold a strong connection. It isn't so much that I am afraid of being struck as that I am afraid of falling and being run over. Not sure my legs can hold me up.

Never thought I'd be grateful for the fat on my stomach, but I am. I've known for years that it protects my vital organs—heart, liver, lungs—from other people's unconscious blasts. (Yes, I've been grateful for that, but always believed if I could protect myself better psychically, I wouldn't need to carry the fat literally.) However, osmosis has always been my body's way of relating—absorbing the atmosphere. Well, now the fat seems to be creating a shield for my lower organs. Where there is a fat shield, I have much less pain. I am taking in light through poetry, music, letters, cards, and flowers. I breathe deep and open to their love, these instruments of the Great cherishing Mother.

"Cast thy bread upon the waters: for thou shalt find it after many days. . . . In the morning sow thy seed, and in the evening withhold not thine hand: for thou knowest not whether shall prosper, either this or that, or whether they both *shall be* alike good" (Ecclesiastes 11:1 and 6).

I am learning the truth, no, I am *experiencing* the truth of these verses.

February 24, 1994

Finished sorting my pictures and slides. Had to use my strong sword of discrimination to sort and let go of so many. The kids laugh at my camera and light meter, but they are my old friends. That camera gave me a way of seeing shapes and colors that is uniquely mine. I remember every frame in the viewfinder before I snapped the shutter. Photographs are meditations for me—like poems.

Luke [Bruce's son] phoned from England. What does one say to these young people who cannot find jobs, have no money, can find no purpose in going on? I remember walking hand in hand with him when he was four. Suddenly he looked up and said, "Why are you so sad?" I was shocked. Neither of us had spoken of sadness. The little boy was fiercely intuitive. The man still is. Luke is a rebel. Life is still very black and very white for him.

Every night I dream of the inner marriage. I, as bride, and my various grooms (a different one every night) are working on the preparations. Whatever the difficulties, no giving up. I wake up every morning feeling cherished and glowing. I have been working very hard, especially with my lawyer and my doctor to encourage my own masculinity to stand up for my femininity. I'm now able to recognize my values *in* a situation (instead of after) and equally able to articulate them.

My dreams are having a powerful effect on our actual marriage. My developing masculinity meets Ross's wit with instant response. He's even falling in love with Ross's femininity all over again. Ross and I are present to each other as never before—concentrating and containing. Our marriage is about separation—moving from fusion to differentiation—moving closer apart.

What we are experiencing is what a Japanese martial arts master once explained to me. What you watch for in your opponent is a *suki*—a moment when his mind goes out of his body. If you are *present*, your conscious mind in your body will know instantly if his conscious mind leaves his body. He is finished once that happens. We aren't sparring, just holding presence. We are accepting the gifts of science that can spare my life immediately; we are also focusing on spiritual and alternative medicines for the future. We're relaxing into the blend of science and soul.

David phoned from Toronto. When I told him about my upcoming two days in the vault, he was silent.

Finally, in a very quiet voice, he said, "Medieval. It's medieval."

"But that's the healing possible for me," I said.

"Maybe you could reframe the idea of the radiation," he said. "Try to concentrate on the creativity of the higher energy."

"That's what I'm trying to do," I said. "I have a sense of that higher energy moving through the leaden slow energy, creating a shift physically and psychically. It's body experience, not intellectual understanding. Balance, David, balance between science and soul."

After I leave the phone, I think more about this hinterland between Earth and Heaven, matter and spirit, archetypal feminine and archetypal masculine. I visualize the radiation as sun radiance permeating my black sapphire. I

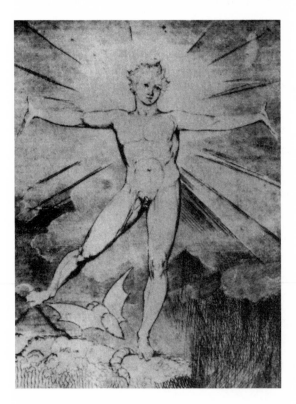

open totally on the breath. I have no idea where the visualization is going. My masculinity is becoming a true Spiritual Warrior— following an unknown path to an unknown goal. He has no alternative. He has nothing to cling to but his trust in the mystery. His armor is his faith; his allegiance is to God/Sophia. All I have to do is let go, cherish him on every step forward and every step back, and leave the rest to Them.

I thank Sophia for all the body work and dream

work I have done in the last twenty-five years—yoga, dance, Feldenkrais, visualization with energy. My soul is consciously present in my cells. My cells are ready to receive high-energy spirit. My own higher vibration is ready to open to an even higher vibration as healer. I can catch a glimpse of myself as a wise Virgin with her lamp ready when the Bridegroom comes.

As I look at my cards so full of love, receive phone calls, look at my flowers, look at Ross, think of my beloved ones, I feel myself embodied in a state of Grace. God is triumphantly with me. Every day—every moment—is a New Day. Dear William Blake—NEW DAY. SPRING. RESUR-RECTION. Forty-eight hours in the tomb, and on the third day I shall rise again—a new woman.

February 26, 1994

Fraser died two years ago.

February 27, 1994

Sunrise! Will I ever forget that radiant Japanese gentleman coming through the French windows into the living room at Esalen with his cello? In broken English he told our group he had a story to tell. Two years earlier he had been diagnosed with cancer with a few months to live. He stopped work. In his musing, he noticed that the birds sang every day in full orchestra twenty minutes before dawn. He

The origin of the word holistic is *holos* in Greek. Some important words derived from *holos* include: whole, heal, health and holy.

—*Shin-ichiro Terayama*

also noticed a particular freshness in the air at that time. He asked his chemist wife what that freshness was. "Oxygen," she said. She brought some home from her lab and in the middle of the night he sprayed a little oxygen into his canary's still-covered cage. The canary began to sing. From that moment he was in his garden every morning twenty minutes before dawn—breathing. His cancer went into remission; he left his heavy job; he took up his cello and now goes around the world telling his story, allowing *Ave Maria* to resonate in the hearts of those who have ears to hear. His delight affirmed my love of the pre-dawn orchestra and the rising sun.

February 28, 1994

Delightful yellow bouquet from Pat—freesias, daffodils, daisies. Spring perfume! Doris [secretary] phoned with her ever-hopeful message. Thank God for her sensation function in my life.

Trying to make realistic decisions re: carpeting and painting in our new condominium. Trying to believe the reality of the move.

Will miss the Olympics. Television is so full of anger, lust, violence, murder one hardly expects to see anything so wholesome and disciplined as these elegant athletes! Dory said the *Globe and Mail* published a big front-page picture of Kurt Browning on his knees on the ice. What is it about Canadians that they highlight failure in their own people? Why do they have to mock each other? Surely this is our shadow—something to do with being fearful of taking first place. We rarely honor with accolades our great dreams and great dreamers. Not that I respect inflation, but I sometimes wonder what we could be if we dared to accept the reality of our fantasies. Has it something to do with never having rebelled against mother and father? And, therefore, despising the rebel child who does go beyond mother and father and the rest of the sleeping collective? In his *Casablanca,* Kurt Browning brought a new sensitivity, new elegance to male skating. Why would the media focus on his fall? Snide, petty stuff—and very dangerous as an undercurrent in our sleepy culture. Perceived and perceiver are one.

March 1, 1994

7:00 A.M.

Looks like March is coming in like a lamb, a cold lamb, but a lamb nonetheless. And with it more snowdrops.

Fearsome dream. Whole city smothered in black vapor. YES, woke up with "Perfect love casteth out fear" (I John 4:18). "Perfect love" is accepting Sophia's love, God's will, and moving into life in full surrender to that love. Archetypally it is turning the negative parents around, claiming the Great Mother and Great Father, thus transforming fear of life into celebration of life. I was actually able to accomplish that surrender in India. I received that love into my cells, let go, trusted whatever was God's will for me. Fearlessly I went into the streets where previously my terror of Death had attracted Death to me—or attracted me into dangerous situations. I moved into teeming life when I let go into Her love reaching out to me through the Indian people.

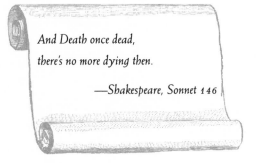

And Death once dead,
there's no more dying then.

—Shakespeare, Sonnet 146

That's all true. But in 1994? The world we are living in is becoming more violent every day. Not only are moral and ethical values becoming obsolete, but drugs can render addicts inhuman. Encounters I used to trust on the streets, I no longer dare because I am no longer sure there is someone at home at the core of a stranger. Nor is there anyone at home at the core of a machine. Rational fear, I think, has to be part of the Spiritual Warrior's armor.

Don't trick yourself into an intellectual cul-de-sac, Marion, or become paranoiac. Your task right now is to let the old thinking go, flush the toilet, accept the love, walk free.

5:00 P.M.

I'm beginning to realize that the radiation is coming to an end. That means that my full responsibility for myself is about to begin. That challenges me. In December I started out with my fresh green and yellow vegetables. I was doing fine until radiation began; then my body felt as if it would explode if I ate one raw carrot. Gave up enzymes for the duration. Finally had to give up emphasis on diet because I had to stay with steamed vegetables, custard, and bananas. Had to give up my reading too. All these splendid books on imagery, diet, and cancer, I could not stay awake to read. Same thing with Zeca's treatment. I just could not agonize over that needle every day. Nor could I get up in the middle of every night to take the right medicine away from food. Even the walks were impossible because the winter knocked my bones into paralytic cold. All the disciplined caring disintegrated. I did what I could to hold the container strong, but now more than that is going to be required. A new regime! Better think New Day because I can rejoice in Blake's New Day. I cannot rejoice in any regime.

Fixed the flowers in our bedroom, on Ross's desk, on the dining room table. Paula phoned. Paula said Mary told her that if I was choosing to go, it was up to her to let me go. She should not stand between me and my destiny. "That's fine for you, Mary Hamilton," Paula said, "but I intend to stand between Marion and her leaving this world until she is clear what is going on." There's real Crone. Paula is older than Mary. One dare not give in to the unconscious drives too soon. The Negative Mother is very, very, very strong on the side of despair in the cells. And it is just a breath from despair to death. Now, the balance between the two snakes in the caduceus has to be absolute. They have to eye each other and be totally alert. If either fails in the concentration, the other strikes and the balance is lost.

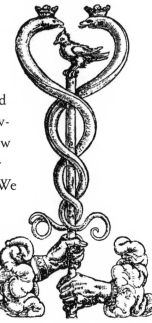

Ross and I are holding that concentration. Neither of us is capable of thinking beyond Saturday. We try to think of Sydenham and moving, but we cannot. The burn is quite serious now with some bleeding. We both feel if we lose our concentration, the counterblow could be fatal. We never said this to each other until today when we were both wondering why we were so unable to act. I did manage to get tickets to England for April. I dream of walking by the sea or on the Devon moors gathering wildflowers in April.

March 2, 1994

Spring sunshine. I am going into the hospital in 1½ hours, so I need to come to grips with my feelings. (That was as far as I got. The phone rang. Nena called.) So much happened so fast that I suddenly found myself putting tapes in my briefcase as quickly as possible with my little Sony, my white buffalo, cards for the shelves, my housecoat and acorns, *Romeo and Juliet*, John Keats's poems, Michael's *The Lost Upland*, Ross's paper on the Inner Meaning of Revelation. Put on my Victorian green, left my mitts because it will be Spring when I come out, gave Ross a strong kiss in the elevator, and we drove through the sunshine to the hospital.

"When we move into the new condo," he said, "it will be Easter Sunday." Easter Sunday and Blake's New Day. We are right in synch.

Put up my cards, fixed the drawers so I could open them without moving my torso. Ross and I checked out the vault. It is small. The lead lining is covered with gray material; all the accoutrements are here for the radiation. One small window that will not open, but at least I can see sunlight. Ross read Keats's poems, especially the ones to his beloved Fanny. I fell in love with my husband yet again. We ate our muffin and drank our Aqua. He dozed. I read Juliet's speech as she prepares to drink the potion that will put her to sleep until she wakes in Romeo's arms.

> *Ah! dearest love, sweet home*
> *of all my fears,*
> *And hopes, and joys, and*
> *panting miseries—*
>
> *—John Keats, "Ode to Fanny"*

> *I have a faint cold fear thrills through my veins,*
> *That almost freezes up the heat of life: . . .*
> *My dismal scene I needs must act alone. . . .*
> *O! if I wake, shall I not be distraught,*
> *Environed with all these hideous fears, . . .*
> *And, in this rage, with some great kinsman's bone,*

As with a club, dash out my desperate brains? . . .
Romeo, I come! this do I drink to thee.

7:15 P.M.

Things began to happen—
ECG, blood samples, blood pressure. Then a long kiss, a chuckle,
and Ross was gone. Difficult
breathing with the sealed window. Giving my soul into
Sophia's keeping and going to
sleep. Well aware most people on this ward are very ill,
most going for surgery tomorrow.

Beloved Sophia,

Give me faith to endure the paradox of life and death. Into your arms I
commend my soul.

—*MW*

March 3, 1994

Awoke with a dream of devastation. Nurses very
friendly. No food or water. Had a shower at the end of the
hall. My phone is broken; phoned Ross from pay phone.
Adrienne had phoned last night, Ursula, and Michele. That
golden web grows stronger.

The orderlies came on schedule. I got on the gurney
myself. The efficient doctors and nurses on the operating
team were kind. Gone from this world in five minutes.

As I come out of the anesthetic, words are sobbing out
of my mouth, "What happened? Whatever happened?" I am
writhing in my abdomen, and my genitals feel as if I've been
raped by an elephant.

"What's wrong?" the nurse asks.

"You have to do something. Now!" I say. "Take that out."

"Pain anesthetizes itself," she says. "Try to hold it for
two hours."

I can't stop begging her to take it out as my teeth chatter with agony. She strokes my forehead and assures me that all will be well. I go back into the anesthetized state and wake up in my vault, ravaged with pain. The big clock on the wall says 12:10. "I'll wait until two," I think.

Can't move, can't write, can't phone. Can speak into my Sony tape recorder.

2:00 P.M.

No relief. The nurses can stay only 45 seconds for fear of their own reproductive systems being radiated. They are doing what they can, but nobody can come close enough to help me. They've placed lead shields around the bed and they don't dare step beyond them. I can't reach the phone. Anyway, it's broken.

4:00 P.M.

No change. Can't reach the drawers. Listen to David Whyte and feel strong reciting with him.

> I was told once, only,
> in a whisper,
> "The blade is so sharp—
> It cuts things together
> —not apart."
>
> (David Whyte, "No One Told Me")

6:10 P.M.

Can endure no longer. Ask the nurse if many people can't take these nodes.

"Most have no problem," she says.

"There's something wrong with the way mine are in," I say.

"I hope not," she says, swinging out of the room after forty seconds. The little girl who brings my supper literally shoves it over the screen and runs. I don't blame her, but I can't reach it. Don't want it anyway.

7:00 P.M.

I ask the nurse to phone the doctor to come and take this out.

"I can't do that," she says.

"Then *I'll* pull it out," I say. "This is not endurable for forty-eight hours."

"You *cannot* do that," she says. "I have orders to give you Demerol."

"Do," I say.

She gives me some; another nurse gives me more. I am drugged, but I keep counting the minutes on the clock. Can't concentrate on David's poetry or Jean's magnificent vision.

March 4, 1994

6:00 A.M.

No bath, no nothing. Thank God the catheter works. Endure for 30 more hours. Someone in the next room cried all night, heartbroken sobbing.

12:00 NOON

Twenty-four hours complete, twenty-four hours to go. I keep praying to Sophia to shield me from these hideous rays, but I can-

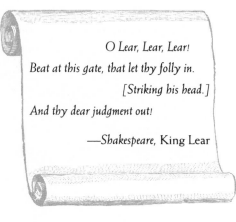

O Lear, Lear, Lear!
Beat at this gate, that let thy folly in.
                    [*Striking his head.*]
And thy dear judgment out!

—*Shakespeare*, King Lear

not concentrate on the prayers. The pain is beyond anything I have ever known. Comes in bolts. If I could concentrate, maybe I could stop the pain. I deep-breathe, try to remain motionless. That works best. See Kathryn and Paul's flowering card. Hold Jill's white buffalo. See Eleanora's two ladies walking by the sea. And dear Mary and John's dying flowers.

4:00 P.M.

With enough Demerol I can be motionless and endure. If only I had Juliet's drink to still my desperate brains!

6:00 P.M.

I tell the nurse I can't go on.
"You can't stop now," she says. More Demerol.

10:00 P.M.

I'm a bit crazy. I signal the nurse to come. Lovely woman. She says she's had her kids, so she'll try to help me for a few minutes. She finds the bed soaked. I don't know why. I only know it's got to end, got to end, end, end. NOW. She throws a new sheet over the shield and pulls the old one while I gently lift up. It is soaked in blood. She can't figure out what's happening. She's sorry she can't stay. I tell her please to get out and care for herself. She gives me a dry pillow and water. The doctors and nurses are doing what they believe to be right, but I cannot believe in my heart that this is good medicine.

March 5, 1994

2:00 A.M.

I read from my little red
Keats book. Writing those great
odes while he coughed his lungs
out! They're different when Death
is real, just at my fingertips.

Greater! Greater! Why would God take
a 26-year-old genius into Death? Nothing makes any sense,
"Here where men sit and hear each other groan." Dear God,
the groaning in these halls and the weeping by both the patients and their families. Every time the door opens in the
night I hear it. More Demerol. Only eight hours to go.

7:00 A.M.

Man comes to turn off radiation tank.

7:15 A.M.

Mercifully a woman doctor whom I have never seen before comes early to take out the nodes.

"What happened here?" she asks as soon as she looks.

"What do you think happened?" I ask, hoping to find
out something.

"Far too much packing," she says, muttering other
things as she pulls packing upon packing out of my vagina,
every piece a torment. "This catheter is going to hurt," she
says. "You're raw." As she pulls, I scream.

OVER. THANK GOD. AND MY ROMEO NOT
DEAD AND ME READY TO GO FREE OF MY VAULT.

8:00 A.M.

Slithered my way along the wall to the bathroom. Very
dizzy, disoriented. Hair matted, body stinking. Bathed.

Found the pay phone. Phoned Ross. He came at once. We came together to Windermere. Resurrection bouquet from Mary Elizabeth. Slept.

April 3, 1994

Unable to do anything for a month after the ordeal. No more cancer. No more radiation. My doctor pronounced me clear on March 29. Felt the crucifixion this year, and the tomb, and Easter Sunday. Still not sure who has emerged.

April 4, 1994

My reserves are so low we canceled England. When we agreed to go a year ago, Ross and I were supposed to teach at Schumacher College in Devon. Memories of England in springtime magnetized us to our beloved haunts. But now the plane ride alone is impossible. Martin advised against it, and Zeca. They said I didn't need any more radiation and the plane provided no cover from the sun's rays. I knew I couldn't cope anyway. Darling Mary took our place. She went off with sweet hope and equal fear.

I walk morning and night. I see the crocuses—so vulnerable, so strong. Their delicate purple and white heads stand up and sing their hosannas in the snow. I become Crocus when I see them. I have to stop and BE with them. My color responses have become so finely tuned I can see

A little Madness in the Spring
Is wholesome even for the King,
But God be with the Clown—
Who ponders this tremendous scene—
This whole Experiment of Green—
As if it were his own!

—Emily Dickinson

gray with a whiff of green becoming more green each day—on the lawn, in the trees. Dear Emily's "Experiment of Green" will soon be here.

Can't help the flying thoughts that wonder if I'll see another spring. Then I become Spring. I become Resurrection—new life, born from the lead vault, my whole body the spiritual womb of creation no longer limited to physical womb. I feel Sophia shudder within me—*quickened*. What a word! *Quickened* in every cell. Desire, love, life— quickened.

At the same time, Ross and I are making an appointment to talk to Needham's Funeral Home about funeral arrangements so neither of us is left trying to make decisions alone when we can't think a thought. The paradoxes become awesome. So awesome we have to postpone the Needham appointment.

April 6, 1994

Took a few boxes of good dishes to Sydenham. Trying to get the feel of that place.

David is working with us in his devoted fashion. He's rebuilt the bookcases and meticulously numbered all Ross's art books so they will go back into the shelves where they came out. He put three coats of almond paint on the kitchen. I want to gently, slowly get all the cupboards set up before we move. Once the innards are in place, the rest follows. Each day I put on the pretty paper and three or more shelves are done. With the stained glass, pendulum crystals with sunbeams flirting on the walls, and my green plants, the kitchen is already very inviting. The accent colors from the pictures are red and rust and the African earthen pots ground the almond.

Ross went to the Baha'i conference in Chicago on March 25. I was glad Sandy could be with him on the train, all the way to and from. This ordeal is horrific for him. He doesn't look well at all, and stress is the worst component for diabetes. I think the powerlessness is even worse for those who have to watch the disease and the treatment.

I stand in my own shoes with Zeca. With him I can ask the right questions and receive sane answers, and make my choices. I am injecting into my thigh every day homeopathic dilutions that are part of his treatment, the other two components I take orally. It gives me strength. I sleep three hours every afternoon, go to bed around eight, and sleep till six or seven. Profoundly tired. Taking good care of my skin where the radiation was. My hair is like hay, but I'll soon cut it off and hope for new curls.

Found this picture taken in my office when John landed in one dark afternoon from London, England.

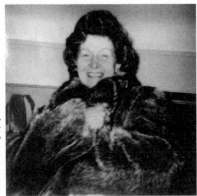

"I want your coat," I said.

"Take it, Marion," he said, and snapped this strong, grounded, gleeful woman that I need to re-member within me.

Dear John, you persisted in your childhood folly and, before you died, had assembled one of the greatest collections of Hollywood stills in the world. Dear, dear John.

May 6, 1994

Ross drove me through spring sunshine to the London Airport. Red tulips hurt—red, so red, so radiantly red. I shakily came to Kripalu, the Yoga center in Massachusetts.

I hadn't felt able to come to this conference. I phoned Stephen to tell him so. "Come here," he said, "even if you can't work. We can take care of you."

"What an extraordinary young man!" I thought.

So to Kripalu on my initiatory journey, moving from the underworld into the sun. I feel very shaky, as if my feet aren't quite on the ground. Had a mean time at customs because I had my hypodermic needles with me. The patriarchal officer heard I was going to the Yoga center and instantly rooted into my bag and found the needles.

"You can take them and throw them out," I said, "but I'm the one who has cancer, and I am dependent on those dilutions."

He gave me a tongue-lashing, and I kept the needles. Small incident, but in my fragile, newborn state of vulnerability, I can't take any kind of confrontation. I feel I have no covering, no protection at all, and no way of judging what to say and what not to say in order to protect myself. I lunge into things, and whatever splats out of my center is there for everyone to deal with. Everything is immediate and often alarming and funny because shocking.

How right Stephen was! And how they can take care of me! I've never experienced anything comparable. One young woman, Meredith, takes care of all my needs, intercedes when people try to hook me into private talks, checks that my food is exactly what I can eat, makes appointments, is present for me in every detail. My room is on the top floor, wide open to the spring breath off the lake.

First, I am given an aromatic facial that begins with a footbath that gradually permeates every cell of my being with sage, juniper, lavender—Cleopatra's spices and warm oils to make her look young when she is old.

The second day, an excellent yoga lesson—private, especially for me in my convalescing state. The teacher is so

cherishing, my body loves her and responds like a child trying to learn its new lessons. I do not find it easy to receive
so much love. I keep wanting to give something back—a
half hour of my time, a book, a walk together—but I no
longer have the energy to give. I have no alternative but to
simply receive. Not easy! Especially when the giving is so
gracious.

Anyway, I feel wonderful after my yoga lesson, right in
tune with my body. Then, as I am putting on my skirt, I
hear coming out of my mouth, "My stomach used to be flat.
It wasn't always flabby like this." Instantly I hear a stricken
voice from inside: "I did my best." Oh dear, oh dear, oh
dear. I hear the cock crow. I start to cry. I am so ashamed of
my betrayal. Truly my dear body has done her very best.
She went through the operation with never a complaint.
She knew the cancer had to come out, and even if it meant
the sacrifice of her womb, she could understand the in-
evitability of loss. She did all she could to accept the discipline of the diet, the rest, the exercise, the pain, yes, the
terror of no longer being whole. And certainly the terror of
the radiation. There were times we stood together at the reception desk and I could hear her saying, "I'm bolting, Marion. I'm not staying." And I would talk to her and we could
go onto the machine together. Then there was the day we
did leave. I knew she was right. We went home for five
days. And then, poor creature, going through the holocaust
of the lead chamber. When my ego was under anesthetic,
she was crying out, "Whatever happened?" She knew something was wrong. Dear God, what a travesty that was—me
drugged out and her being radiated, burned—whatever
horror was going on there—and no consciousness at all
doing anything about it. No phone—nothing! And after all
that, to betray her. To swing into collective values, values
that have destroyed my health for almost fifty years, and in

a throwaway moment to throw her away! When will I learn? Thank God I was able to cry.

I came back to my room and sobbed and begged Sophia's forgiveness. She pulled me right into her lap, and we slept in her loving arms.

May 7, 1994

That centering made my lecture possible. I had felt very fearful that nothing would form in my head or come out of my mouth. However, Saturday morning did come, and with it my energy began to reach out to an audience once again. The wave of love that came back to me was so strong that I melted into it and spoke straight from heart in the moment. It was good to try again, but I left exhausted.

May 11, 1994

Did my fingernails, worked on my hair, tried to put sentences together in my head—in short, tried to bring my body into consciousness and my mind. My heart rarely fails me. Went to Sleeping Giant TV productions, talked with Rita [TV interviewer] for almost five hours. Everyone was very happy as the program progressed. It is strange to have strangers so pleased when I am just being myself. Strange too to hear things coming out of my mouth I didn't know were in my realization before, and in a deep rich voice that comes straight from center. It is good, I think, to try to move out into the world again. I worry that I am going out too soon, that I am too tired when the shootings are over. But I am so deep into myself I don't want to come out and I could fall away from society totally. And I could fall into no language, no consciousness. I need to hold the tension of the opposites.

Had excellent sessions with Zeca and Helga. The office is full of music and tangerine essence. My body relaxes into being cared for, being loved. No more needles!

May 18, 1994

Back to my oasis in the studio. What freedom to shut that door and be alone. I love Ross, I love people, but I can't keep up anymore. I need to be able to melt away. I melt into ivory orange blossoms, new robins—the eggs that fly off in music (Emily Dickinson)—the purple finch that greets me every morning at four-thirty and sits on the balcony, chatting and singing, while I write.

May 19, 1994——Royal York Hotel

Again pulling myself together for a conference. Actually put on black pants and my big white shirt. Feel quite sexy, although I'm not in sexual gear right now. Terribly nervous. What if I just want to watch instead of engage? What if my introvert wants to hide in the bathtub and won't come out? What if the old chemistry won't work anymore in the sessions with Robert? What if my energy is no longer big enough to meet his?

How I remember coming into Toronto on the train from London to go to the College of Education, my suitcases full of cookies and jams and fruitcakes from Mother's kitchen. How I gazed at the biggest hotel in town and wondered if I might one day spend my honeymoon in the Royal

York! Zenith of elegance! So here it is, Bubbles. You're on! You're speaking in the Royal York.

Registered with no sense of being here. Came upstairs. Great room—chintz, king-size bed, big bathtub long enough to lie flat in, gold fixtures, and unguents to be smoothed on soft skin, and piles of white towels. Instantly my circuit began to pump adrenaline. Downstairs to the underground mall to buy fruit and tulips to make my room home. Free, now, free. Free to dance to my music, dream in my tub, come and go as I please with this place as center. Love the mall—haven't been in such pollution for six months. Bought fingernail polish, eye shadow, cream and black panty hose. Let my shadow play around the food shops, found where I want to have breakfast.

Realized with a crash I was on for a full-day session tomorrow. Suddenly started coughing and feeling very hot. Robert arrived with his great arms open, and I knew if I couldn't sustain it, he could. He chuckles a lot more than he used to, just a joyous overflow.

May 20, 1994

Great sessions with 150 people on our video series *On Men and Women*. As Robert and I sat at the back watching it, both of us were periodically swept by embarrassment. Interchanges, insights were lost that we both see as crucial now. Feel so vulnerable with no way to change what is encapsulated in film. The audience was so loving we totally relaxed into it.

Evening opening of conference very difficult. Too tired. Ballroom too big. Didn't feel myself there. Felt like a naked baby bird thrown out of the nest. Saw my dear friends in the audience, but I wanted to be Hans Hedgehog and crawl away to my den.

May 21, 1994

Robert went to his son's graduation in Minnesota, so John and I carried on. I feel so grounded. I don't say anything that doesn't come straight off my tongue. Result is riveting. Had trouble in the men's session today; many of them I've worked with at conferences for years.

I said, "I don't want to be Mother for you anymore. I do not want to carry that projection."

Rebellion. "That's who you are. That's who you've always been. That can't be changed."

"Well, it can be," I said. "I am not there anymore."

I could feel anger in the room and I felt threatened because I knew I could be their adored Mother just by turning the sentence around. I assured them I didn't want to keep them as boys. Time for them to grow up. Much, much unresolved anger in that session.

Robert back for Saturday night. Coleman reading Rumi and his own poetry in his flat southern drawl—fabulous! Great bear of a man with all those antennae. So is Robert. His body picks up every rhythm, every nuance of feeling. People mock him for his body response to poetry. How they should envy him for his aliveness to its vitality. David looking luminous with his sitar, playing exquisitely. And Marcus in full command with his tabla, utterly sensitive in his soul. Doug superb—ready at every moment with a poem or a song or a shocking laugh. He's a *real* clown. In the moment, absolutely in the moment. What a privilege to be with these men, to love and be loved by them as precious friends.

Mary is magnificent. Her body sessions are right on, superbly aligning body, mind, spirit. Mel and Shirley from Winnipeg bring genuine native American strength and purity of intent.

I'm gradually moving in. Thank you, Sophia. For a while I thought I might go home and never dare a conference again.

May 22, 1994

Sunday—everything in place with Robert back. One of the men told me of a complaint in the men's group over my not being Mother anymore. Robert replied, "She's woman first. You have to accept that." "You've got it right, Robert," I said to myself. We had a big argument onstage. It was as if each of us had to work new insights through to mutual understanding. I could feel my rumbling energy rally itself to meet his. The dynamic was as intense as ever—energetic respect.

One thing I learned yet again is the power of nature to heal. I knew there was no nature in the Royal York. I also knew that the closing ritual of sacrifice and purification could not work if participants weren't met in love as they left the ceremonial room. In other venues they walked out and the healing that began inside was carried through by trees and rocks. In the Royal York they walked out the inner doors of the ballroom and were met by pillars and crystal chandeliers. What happened? Most of them collapsed on the floor beside the pillars, sobbing or staring into space. The upstairs foyer

> The soul is not in the body; the body is in the soul.
>
> —*Hildegard von Bingen*

looked as if someone had just been through with a machine gun and sounded like it too. Nature was not there to enfold her children. Some of us did our best to greet their tender souls, but I saw how utterly the Great Mother does her job with grass and trees and water. We are too often unconscious of the great gift we are in.

Left the hotel with Mary. Caught the Via train to London. John had made first-class reservations for us, so against all rules for curing cancer we sat eating and laughing and drinking wine all the way home. Couldn't believe we were in London. Couldn't walk straight off the train either. Or fly.

May 24, 1994

Our precious old pear tree, her skeleton quite black, is dancing in her wedding dress in our spring garden. To the clinic. Didn't see my doctor, but everything seems fine except for digestion problems. Still quite dependent on Ultra-Clear Sustain once a day at least. Feel my body close down as soon as the hospital is in sight. That was not so before the weekend of the lead vault.

May 27, 1994

Lectured all day to social workers at University Hospital. Some of my students from 30 years ago were there. Felt good to be completing a circle. Wore white pants and tangerine shirt and white shoes. For some reason the white shoes took on a life of their own and I felt them dancing around on the floor beneath me—doing a soft shoe. They actually were living their fun while I talked. I was so happy to have the chalk in my hand again. Greg mentioned this phenomenon to Ross. He said I was totally embodied, seemed to be dancing the whole time I was lecturing. My teaching life was resurrected.

I was very happy, but very tired. When I talked to Mary, she said she saw me dance down the ballroom in the Royal York—my spirit flying through the air, my body too tired to walk, let alone fly. Have to watch this. I know she is right. This separation is what has caused my sickness. The two vibrations do not meet in unison.

May 28, 1994

Ross and Mary and I slipped off to Toronto in the dark on the Robert Q [airbus]; to the West Coast, Cortez Island, and Holly-hock Farm on Air Canada. Life is coming back into me. I feel the adventure of ferrying from one island to another, trying to find the next ride while crossing on the ferry.

> Or like stout Cortez when
>   with eagle eyes
> He stared at the Pacific—and
>   all his men
> Looked at each other with a
>   wild surmise—
> Silent, upon a peak in Darien.
>
> —John Keats,
> "On First Looking into
> Chapman's Homer"

Whole chest opens to the ocean and the forested hills, the silent mountains majestic in the background. Why would anyone live anywhere else in Canada except on these gulf islands? In my slightly disoriented state—never quite sure feet and head are together—I really feel like Cortez: We have journeyed to some foreign hideaway on the edge of nowhere. Terrible storm as we came. Now sunshine abundant.

June 8, 1994

Two excellent workshops during the week—honest, intense. Ross and Mary and I walked miles by the ocean in the mornings and at noon, felt health pouring into our lungs. This whole week turned out to be—for Ross, especially, in a way we could never have anticipated—a healing. The cancer has undermined him just as much as myself. Now he feels the flesh-and-blood world can be dealt with.

Mary and I worked in 99 percent harmony. We had one round of clashing wills. I was trying to lift my suitcase. She roared, "Marion, put that case down. That's stupid."

"I'm not Gandolf," I said. (She always refers to Gandolf, her big retriever buffoon, as stupid.)

As we faced each other head-on, a man in a truck waiting to move onto the ferry jumped out, grabbed the case in question, and we all jumped into his cab. I find it very difficult being unable to carry my own load. But inside, I know I can't carry that case any farther. I think I carried my part of the workshop very well. I didn't try to do anything extra. Trying to stop mothering and develop my sword of discretion. All my dreams make that clear.

July 7, 1994

The moving van arrived before 8:00 A.M. We had to rush to keep up with the four men carrying the stuff out. They were totally disciplined. With all the work we had done transporting books and dishes and treasured objects, they had everything out by noon. I couldn't believe the speed and efficiency with which one leaves a world once things move into motion. We slept in our gray bedroom for the first time, the soft evening breeze blowing through from Bob's fragrant garden below. It was like old times in the parsonage, big rooms, high ceilings, broad windows. We feel somewhat overwhelmed by such generous space.

A little oasis—this *Virgin Ouverente!* The Great Mother contains in her womb all the Christian activity. She is the holder of it all—God the father, who in turn holds his crucified son within his womb. The saints looking on can see only the male relationship. They can't realize that they themselves are held within the container of the Mother. The doors of entry are Her very body. Looked at strictly objectively, how strange this Christian religion is! The sleepy, somewhat perplexed old father lovingly allows his only incarnated son to be crucified, hung there at the crux between Heaven and Earth, Spirit and Matter, to redeem the sins of the world. In this image the activity is all hidden within Her womb.

I try not to speak about my fear that this move is all too much for both of us separately and together. We try to have our sleep every afternoon, try to keep a good diet of green and yellow vegetables, try to walk every evening. Together we are moving slowly, steadily, and with great delight in our new playhouse.

We are both using the *concentration* we noted in Fran and Dave's house. We work on a room a day. One picture on each wall, exactly hung. No extra objects. All vistas are kept clear from every direction. Repeatedly I am surprised by joy when I see the beloved objects looking so new and so elegant in their new location. The colors of the rooms are perfect for our goods and chattels.

I had measured exactly where I hoped my furniture would go when it came from Toronto for my new office here. To my surprise, it worked. Need a celadon green cover for the couch, need my stained glass in place on the windows, some warmth around the fireplace, and we're set.

The passivity of some of the craftsmen who come to work with us is alarming. Ross and I are not trained to make a house burglarproof. We bring in the "experts," they dawdle their way around and wait for us to tell them what to do. We don't know! The ironmonger measured the doors and windows for bars. When he finished, I saw the stained glass window utterly vulnerable from above. I asked him about it and he said, "I'd certainly want that protected. Anyone could climb off the roof." Same thing with the kitchen—the most vulnerable window never measured. Passive aggression is the opposite of creativity. Same attitude we found thirty years ago in England when we were trying to fix our Baby Belling—that crazy tiny stove. We didn't think that "can't help it" attitude would ever come here. Well, it has. The chimney men half looked at the fireplace and chimney, didn't check for raccoon holes and squirrel nests, took their eighty dollars, and left. Within an hour, I was enjoying a telephone chat, felt a thud on my head, and beheld a squirrel on the kitchen stove!

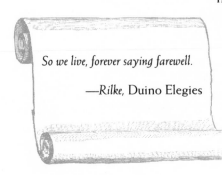

So we live, forever saying farewell.

—*Rilke*, Duino Elegies

In the midst of all this Jeffrey [friend] died a terrible death from AIDS. His rage against the collapsing culture was devastating. His love of language, books, theater was continually barraged. His passion was in league with Lucifer—the light bearer—and equally conflicted. Kill the King; long may I reign.

August 1, 1994

Felt pain in my back. Trying to sit straight without crossing legs, trying to walk straight without dragging left leg, but I'm not in balance and can't be because putting that foot squarely on the ground is hell in my hips. Try to walk an hour every day but often have to rest on the grass before coming home.

August 8, 1994

Now Bruce's arrival. Ross told him on the phone he had to come. We have to have him. Bruce knows exactly how to do things in caring for a house. He has just finished putting Holmesdale [his home in England] into 100 percent condition for selling. So, so glad to see him. Almost instantly he was through the back gate and through the parking lot on his way to the hardware a block away. Like Father and Fraser, he believes in making good friends with the hardware merchant. And he loves running to the shops for treats, the morning paper, people. No one had been through our back gate until he arrived. In fact, I wanted to seal it off. No way! He's out through that space five times a day. He instantly bought hammer, special nails, garden snips, fertilizer, bird feeder. We always have a good talk in the morning (6–7) and then Ross gets up and we start our project for the day. Actually Ross and I were doing all we could to get the place together before Bruce came—and we do have the character of every room established, paintings and furniture in position—but now real problems are presenting themselves. And, thank God, Bruce is here because we would be throwing good money after bad not knowing what to do or where to find the right workman.

Our window armatures would not work. We had them fixed. But Bruce took one look and said, "They'll never work. The sills are full of wood lice." He poured turpentine on them and out poured the lice. So new window ledges throughout. And so on to new windows. Old vine fittings torn off the house, the arbor pulled down, reconstruction of the garden (love the great V shapes he created), keys to fit all doors. Every day some new task about heat or air conditioning, chimney, squirrels or bats is dealt with. We're gradually feeling we're here. Even the CD player works now, and all the automatic switches on the lights.

But Ross is getting thinner and whiter and more distracted every day. He seems withdrawn, holding something that can explode.

August 15, 1994

Celebrated my birthday together all three. My annual birthday poem from Ross.

THE READINESS IS ALL

It is hardly a cause for celebration.
I mean the year with all its grief,
The leaden weight of closing down.

You who came rejoicing
With your healing, dancing eyes,

And the eager, deliberate stride
That brought newness to the day,
The sense of a fresh beginning
In a world that is always now.

None of this is gone. A flower greets you,
A card from Bruce, the bicycle painted white,
Daisies in a new arrangement,
A sense of where things belong,
And the love with which they're brought there,
There where the Buddha sleeps.
Oh, the concentrated placing,
The soul in-gathered and still.
The heart in hiding opens
To a world that none can see,
Save those who still can look
Into the depths of your eyes
And steady themselves in your gaze
That draws their infinite sadness in
To a place where they are known:
Neither judged, nor forgiven, but known.
"This is the way things are. This it has always been."
Acceptance is all that remains.

As always, he strikes into the already presence of where
we are right now. Poignant and powerful. He also had my
beloved Sheaffer pen reconstructed so I feel again the one
line through my life. And one glowing sunflower. Precious
gifts, precious man!

Bruce painted my stationary bicycle (which he gave
Mother 20 years ago, still in excellent shape) and put a big
red bow on it. He bought my once-a-year butter pecan ice
cream. Luscious!

Went to Springbank—eternal Springbank—for a long walk. Ate popcorn, watched the kids on the merry-go-round that we once loved. Quiet, sylvan London.

Focused effort with our trees—pruned half the pear trees away, half the apple and shaped the two mountain ash. Four squirrels' nests went, leaving at least one crazed squirrel, who took to chasing robins in the back garden, running over them so they temporarily couldn't fly. All our hedges are now shaped—fundamental cutting for next year.

August 16, 1994

Paul arrived. Paul with his two uncles was very much a man. He put his stamp of approval on our home, laughed at how the electricity was wired, laughed at the heating organization—but loved the place. Ross looks so unwell we are all worried. Paul finally said, "Look, Uncle, I'm going to carry you to the island if I have to." Ross and I are very uncertain about getting too far away from the hospital because he had a strange experience in the night when that energy bolt came up out of his belly through his neck, behind his left eye and exploded. Dr. Cohen thought it was a stroke. So did the doctors in emergency at St. Jo's—but no residual symptoms. With Paul here there is nothing to worry about in preparing the island. Together we decided to entrust ShaSha [Island] with his health.

August 17, 1994

Bruce and Paul drove to Toronto. Ross lay in the front seat of our Camray and I drove to Barrie to pick up the younger generation.

ShaSha never changes. Sophia bless her. Whatever hell is going on outside, ShaSha IS. We settled into three halcyon days with Marion and Aidan, Paul, Kathryn and Marion Rose, and Siobhan [niece from England]. Some problems between the babies because Aidan in his love for Marion bites her. This causes problems between the mothers. Kathryn has had a hard trimester in her second pregnancy, so she isn't seeing much fun in anything. Ross and I are arms-wide-open grateful for the fresh air, the wide expanse, the forever beauty.

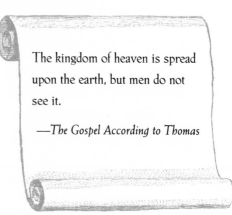

The kingdom of heaven is spread upon the earth, but men do not see it.

—*The Gospel According to Thomas*

August 18, 1994

On ShaSha, the birds sing their saddest songs in late August. I listen. I remember the mornings at dawn, 4:00 A.M., opening my arms to the rising sun and singing "Unto the hills" while the young osprey squawked. Remember running over the rocks from the Teahouse to Miranda [cottage]. Fresh coffee. Settling in to write. Musing with the dark blue fading from the sky as the apricot took over. Watching the Arctic loons playing in puddles of pink in the bay. A beaver or otter or mink diving near the rocks. Climbing through all the mansions of ShaSha with our beloved friends. This year I couldn't move out of Miranda alone. Finally I said I was going to Mount Sinai if I died on the way. I didn't. And I didn't fall. The whole of God's great creation was there.

August 19, 1994

Drove the families to the marina in Parry Sound. Ross and I decided to stay on with Siobhan. (Bruce now in Winnipeg at the opening of his movie *For the Moment*.)

Siobhan is an angel, an exquisite angel, come to live with us for a few days. She gently, firmly moves about the rocks, the patio, the cabin, bringing healing to Ross. She has devoted herself to bringing him back to life by reading poetry to him and having him read to her twenty-four hours a day if necessary. She senses that he cannot live without imagery, and she is determined to resurrect his soul along with her own. She's worked for too many years in a corporation. She adores him and he adores her. They sit out on the patio together hour by hour in the sunshine, sometimes a swim, sometimes a juice, then back to the beloved poems.

August 21, 1994

As we're about to have lunch, Ross decides to read "Sailing to Byzantium." Without quite realizing where the poem is taking us, he reads,

> *An agéd man is but a paltry thing,*
> *A tattered coat upon a stick, unless*
> *Soul clap its hands and sing, and louder sing*
> *For every tatter in its mortal dress.*
>
> (*William Butler Yeats, "Sailing to Byzantium*)

We all three weep. He is that agéd man; he is so thin his tattered clothes hang upon his small frame. And there he is reading his beloved poetry—at last his soul clapping and singing—and louder singing for every tatter—every heartache, every overwhelming anxiety of this horrendous summer, this horrendous year, this horrendous mortality. His soul is back and somehow we are sailing back into life. Siobhan says, "Maybe we should leave this afternoon." Ross and I look at each other surprised. "Yes," we agree.

We sweep, clean, pack, turn off hydro and water in Miranda and the Teahouse. We do our rituals of thanksgiving and good-bye with the rocks and the trees as we return ShaSha to Nature for the winter. Ross and Siobhan bring *Pegasus* [boat] from Iris Bay, we pile everything in, take the garbage to the dump, say good-bye to the bears, and drive through the waves to Parry Sound. I sing my hymns as loud as I can in the stern of the boat. Ross is human again.

August 24, 1994

An attack of agony like I've never had before in that same place in the left side of my lower spine and sacrum. I can't stand, sit, lie without tears pouring out of my eyes. I think of Sonja and Fraser. Is this where I too am to end? After a day of realizing that no heating pad, no hot-water bottle, no nothing can stop the pain, I go to Dr. Cohen and she gives me anti-inflammatories. Just as she hands me the prescription, she says, "You could buy a walker, you know."

"Walker?" I say, not believing my ears. "Me? Walker?"

LEAR: *O me! My heart, my rising heart! but down!*

FOOL: *Cry to it, nuncle, as the cockney did to the eels when she put 'em i' th' paste alive; she knapp'd 'em on th' coxcombs with a stick, and cried, "Down, wantons, down!"*

—*Shakespeare*, King Lear

"Yes," she says, "you'll need it in six months and you might as well learn to use it while you can still walk. Your back is full of osteoarthritis."

I thank her for the suggestion and decide to walk an hour every day no matter what the pain. Just moving the muscles will bring calcium into the bone. Still, I don't want to destroy my spine completely by writhing in pain that may be doing incalculable damage to my nerve centers.

August 25, 1994

Dr. Cohen's anti-inflammatories are miracle drugs. One dose and I got up in the night and realized I could walk with no pain. Took the anti-inflammatories yesterday, then this morning my stool is full of blood. That chills me to the bone. The first question my oncologist always asks is, "No blood in the stool?" "CANCER!" I think. Call Dr. Cohen, say I am going off anti-inflammatories until I know what is going on with the blood. She tells me to come to her office. I do. We make an appointment for a bone scan, the week after I return from Abraxas.

September 2, 1994

Bruce stayed at the studio hoping for some work. No luck! I am going to Abraxas to do a seven-day workshop with Mary, Ann, and Paula. Don't want to leave Ross alone, so Bruce came to London. I think one of our biggest problems in this condo is its size and our age. It is so big we don't hear each other from room to room. We are used to living within breathing range of each other, knowing what each is doing just by the sound, even by the presence in the other room. At Windermere I could always hear his television and know where he was psychically when I went into his space. Or feel his concentration with his computer. Now that connection is gone. I enter his space cold, as he enters mine. If he calls to me, often I don't hear him. And vice versa. Unless we check, we often think the other is ignoring us or we get the message wrong. It is very hard. It is like living alone in big, uninhabited rooms. We've both shrunk out of our own presence and don't fill the space. The hall from his study to mine is longer than the 401 highway. We're like two shadows that eat together, sleep together, but have no substance to relate to each other. We both feel we took on too much. I think we're both fearful for the future.

> Maturity: loving without losing identity.
>
> —MW

September 3, 1994

Abraxas! Difficult balancing act. Mary, Ann, and I had the old fun of riding in Mary's van through golden rich Ontario farmland to Orangeville. There we had a very poor lunch. Our sentimental love of "old country food" landed us with overcooked everything. Disgruntled, we drove on to Abraxas, cradled in the Caledon Hills. So at home seeing the barn—our sacred space. Instantly think of dreams from last year, incidents in body work and voice sessions, and the splendid masks that integrate the work. Think of the courageous women who dare this transformative process.

My body was looking forward to the hot tub and the pool and nervous about everything else, nervous because I foresee a big shift in leadership dynamics. I know I do not have the physical strength to do what I once did in terms of personal work. I know I have to defend myself against unconscious Negative Mother projections, have to rest, have to be very disciplined with food, and most of all have to find a place of leadership which is no longer archetypal Great Mother. And I have to do that before the negative projection sets in when I fail to open up the boundless energy I no longer have.

The ladies are more than gracious in receiving me. They are truly delighted to welcome me back from the dead. I know their prayers have been with me all year, and I tell them how grateful I am for that intricate golden net that goes all over America with its tiny lights of love. Many of them have imaged it that way as well.

Mary has added administration to her workload. Ann is staying steady with her voice and mask work. Paula is the one I worry about because although she is priceless as container in the workshop, I know her role is not sufficiently defined.

September 4, 1994

Made it clear today that I cannot do any personal interviewing and may not appear in the evenings. Talked about having cancer, what the winter has been like, and how I now feel very ambivalent about being here at all. Talked about my sense of nakedness, of being in another dimension, of coming from stark truth, which isn't necessarily easy for them. Talked about feeling myself in liminal space—neither in the past, which I have left with the closing of my Toronto office and basic withdrawal from the lecture circuit, nor in the future, which might be fundamentally writing, introversion, essentially alone with God.

Part of me doesn't want to speak at all and part is hyper in being with people again.

Mary, Ann, Paula, and I guide the workshop from my room overlooking the meadow, meeting morning, noon, and night. Usually we enjoy supper downstairs with the group.

September 5, 1994

The voice becomes louder inside me: "You aren't pulling your own weight. Really no purpose in being here. Stop while the party's in full sun. Don't toddle into twilight." This voice is beginning to undermine me because I can't find my balance when I walk. I need someone's arm. I have to sit when I teach. I experience myself as awkward, not together, arms and legs not coordinated. Sometimes I even feel drunk, unable to control my lower limbs. Never before, however big or small, have I felt myself awkward. Part of me feels like going home.

A certain irony in all of this because we are working on the masculine in women and my very bones are frail, although I have been exercising all summer and eating well. On some of our night walks (Bruce, Ross, and I) I remember trying to hold my back still with my hands to avoid blinding pain when I put my foot down. Remember having to sit in wooden chairs only, not even the luxury of padded, hard upholstery. Little things that I did to protect myself in the summer—things I took no notice of then—are suddenly becoming noticeable. Now I am *trying* to go into the hot tub, *trying* to walk alone across the lawn, *trying* to walk at all on uneven ground. That's how I'm exercising my masculine assertiveness these days! To top my courage off, my Warrior brought the anti-inflammatories just in case!

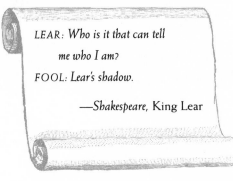

September 6, 1994

Abraxas does not help my stress level. I experience myself as totally different but not quite sure how. Never sure what's going to come out of my mouth. Try to be absolutely straightforward, even after, especially after, I have shocked the women by the sharpness of cutting off old mothering instincts that would sap my energies and keep them infantile.

Love the whirlpool. Keeps me infantile!

September 8, 1994

Mary and I are having a transitional time. She is trying to mother me: "Go to bed. Don't come down here at night. Rest in the afternoon." I know she's right. I do my best to take care, but I need to keep my fingers on the pulse of the workshop too. Otherwise I should be home. If I can't do it right, I don't want to be here. But what is right now? Maybe what I have to offer right now is the teaching, period! But I cannot teach without the feeling tone being right, and that cannot be right if I am not seeing their pictures, hearing their images, watching their bodies.

This morning I was talking to Paula and broke down crying, "I don't feel I'm able to pull my own weight." That shocked me. "The Queen is dead. Long live the Queen," I said, even more shocked. That stopped Paula and Mary and Ann. They may have vulnerability issues, but they assume I will be steady. When I start to crumble at the top, where is their empowerment? What is their reaction to my weakness? How do we become peers? Much unresolved. We'll let Sophia guide us. All will happen as it should at the right time—*kairos*.

September 16, 1994

Went to clinic for bone scan. Asked the technician, "What's this for?"

"Don't you know?" he roared at me.

"I'm not deaf," I said. "I asked you a civil question. What I want to know is whether a bone scan can detect cancer cells or does it just detect abnormality."

"Abnormality," he said.

But the feeling was destroyed. He had to treat me as a stupid, old woman that he could pummel or a smart-ass professional who asked too many questions. At the desk the other day, Lucille asked my name, and when I gave it, the woman and the man who were writing behind looked up. Lucille said, "Oh, you're the one who asks so many questions!" I didn't respond.

Trying to do a few interviews by phone just to give me a sense of doing something worthwhile, but may be exhausting myself with no focused purpose of my own. Until I get that focus, I think I should rest and walk, eat right, and meditate—my fourfold path.

September 19, 1994

To University Hospital for a mammogram. Feel no worry there, no sense of breast cancer. Feel no real worry with the bone scan either. Got the reading on that today—severe degenerative osteoarthritis. Dr. Cohen will send it to my doctor just to make sure it is clear of cancer.

September 21, 1994

To Williamsburg, Virginia. To Eleanora's first. My trips are really to see new places, visit old friends. Missed Eleanora so much this year at ShaSha. We love to lie under the stars and talk and talk and talk. She too has had knee trouble, cannot dance now. Sad when I saw the pictures of her, so exquisitely dressed, so proud, so into the competition with her handsome partner. Felt instantly into those pictures. Felt twenty-five, finding my own glamorous self. I was tango. I was waltz. I was Charleston. Oh, Lord, no need to worry about my body when I could dance three nights a week, every cell resonating. My partners thought I was in love with them. But it was the fantasy of love, the sheer transcendence of movement and music. I became spirit. There's a paradox—the ecstasy of body releasing into spirit.

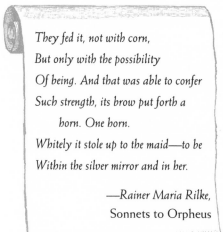

They fed it, not with corn,
But only with the possibility
Of being. And that was able to confer
Such strength, its brow put forth a
    horn. One horn.
Whitely it stole up to the maid—to be
Within the silver mirror and in her.

—Rainer Maria Rilke,
Sonnets to Orpheus

September 22, 1994

Eleanora and I walked for two hours by the sea—rough, turbulent, the tide forcing its way in, wave upon heavy wave. We walked as close to it as we could, using real strength through the wet sand. So invigorated by the wind and water splashing up to our knees. The elements demanded everything.

Had an Alexander treatment. Felt good to feel that central core holding me again. My body has felt so disharmonious, yet I can't do the exercises I need to re-create harmony.

Eleanora, Cliff, and I went to Williamsburg this afternoon. The film on the Revolution made me aware of the deep conflict in the settlers who wanted to stay with England yet knew they had to be free. I never thought about the personal side of that before. Never before thought about the depth of loyalty in my United Empire Loyalist ancestors who gave up everything in Pennsylvania, sailed across Lake Ontario, landed with nothing but their integrity on the bleak coast of Canada. Wasp Canadians do have a very different heritage from Americans. We were the homesick courageous children; they were the courageous rebels.

Went to the battlefield, through the houses, to the hotel with its revolutionary menu, girls singing and playing violins, candles in old sticks. Real sense of the dignity of old Williamsburg.

September 23, 1994

Graciela was here to meet me at the hotel. She came all this way to give me one of her incredible treatments. So glad to see her, so glad to feel her hands ready to touch my back. She had a companion with her to ground my feet. They brought light food. Won't have to worry about meals for the whole weekend.

Very uncertain being with strangers again, realize I am veiled but can't take off the veil and know I need it. People are most kind, but I can't come full out or fully let them in.

The hotel is the Hilton, but the bed is so rocky I had to put the mattress on the floor. Carpet stank of phenol, so I filled up with phlegm. My eyes became very teary and I realized I need to cry. Graciela is bringing up my body grief in the loss of my feminine organs, and terror around the pain in my back. She is also putting me into deep relaxation, total letting go that doesn't seem quite appropriate since I am a speaker. Still, I trust. If deeper healing is to happen, deeper surrender is necessary.

September 24, 1994

Graciela's second treatment took me deeper than the first. She does not think I have cancer, but she does think I have a long way back to Earth. I felt bereft after she left—unprotected, fearful. Although I am surrounded by southern hospitality, I have to put a barrier between me and it. I feel myself in danger of loss of soul simply because I am so vulnerable. The folks only mean to be kind. I know that, but I also know my frailty, and my capacity to compensate by giving all.

September 25, 1994

Thoroughly enjoyed the other speakers. This morning dear Robert Johnson said the whole thing was "Words, words, words—time to put an end to words." I agreed totally, all the time feeling the energy draining out of my body in response to "put an end to words." I knew I had to *speak* this afternoon. I had no words. I couldn't speak. Felt overcome with loneliness.

When I went into the foyer, Greg, ever on the right spot at the right time, said, "What is wrong with you? You are so white."

"Don't know," I said, no longer bereft. "I'll rest."

Went to my room and prayed, clarified the literal and symbolic worlds. Pulled myself into Sophia's loving arms, dressed, and went to speak. My energy wasn't totally in, but as soon as I stood up and saw those loving faces, I could feel myself coming to center. By which I mean I could feel my ego surrendering to God/Sophia, surrendering to their love. I no longer feared forgetting words or gaps in concentration. No longer feared blathering empty words. No longer feared I might drop from loss of energy. No longer feared. I knew what was present in me was totally trustworthy. And it was! Had a humorous, sad, no-frills contact with the audience. Loved the closing dance. Came back to Toronto.

September 28, 1994

Three days in Toronto completing closing rituals with analysands. Delighted to see them again, glad to feel them leaving the nest, flying away on their own wings. Making the boundaries clear is important to their release and my release. Again awed by the *isness* of soul meeting soul in the spaceless, timeless world where essence is all. Told them about Ross in the Arctic selecting Inuit sculpture. He had walked behind a guide through a blizzard carrying an armful of drawings. The guide arrived at the door of the hut ahead of Ross, heaved the door open against the wind, let it slam shut behind him. Ross had to drop some of his rolls in order to pull the door open. Later when he commented on how he had been treated by the guide, he was told that if an Inuit dislikes you he cares for you in a storm, makes you dependent. If he likes you, he allows you your independence. That in the Arctic can mean your survival.

Definition. Differentiation. Distinction. Good masculine attributes! Paradoxically, I am aware of maturing masculine energy releasing more of my femininity out of the Mother archetype and into the Virgin, who is standing to her own hard-won values and feelings, however vulnerable she seems.

October 1, 1994

Preparing to fly to Winnipeg to do Grand Rounds at St. Boniface Hospital. Thinking about the difference between healing and curing. "To Cure or to Heal? The Role of Love in Becoming Whole." (The subtitle was not advertised.) Curing is saving the body from death. Healing is bringing the individual to wholeness. Will speak of my own experience. I've nothing to lose. I will not be discouraged when the doctors tell me that dreams are purely anecdotal, impossible to prove anything from dreams. Nor will I hesitate when I see their discomfiture when I use the word "love." And when I see them looking at the clock, I will quietly proceed with my examples of metaphor as the healing bridge between psyche and soma. And when they afterward shake my hand and say, "That is beautiful poetry," I will smile graciously and remember my verse from the

I will set my face to the wind and scatter my handful of seeds on high.

—*The Koran*

Koran. This is a different Grand Rounds from what I have done before because now I am a cancer patient and I am speaking from my bones.

Dr. Thomas may *cure* my cancer, but he does not want to be aware of my soul. For him, wholeness, *healing* as I understand it, does not exist. I know Zeca and Helga have brought me healing through their love, and sensitivity, and remedies. I know they believe I will get well, and their faith gives me strength to stay with my diet, my walking, my meditation. When they talk to me, I experience myself as myself—seen, heard, touched. I walk out of their office feeling whole. Even if I died of a heart attack in the street, I would die healed. I don't think I would be alive now without Zeca and Helga. When I went to them last December, I was so sick I could barely pull myself up the stairs and I had forgotten I was anybody. Zeca sometimes plays well-orchestrated children's music when I'm there—"When You Wish upon a Star," for example. Of course it brings up Mara and Marion Rose and Aidan for me, but it also ignites my own fresh wonder at the new world in which I find myself. I am a child again, but this time, a conscious child. Higher innocence!

Suddenly I am very angry when I think of being minimized by being told I speak in beautiful poetry. There's an unspoken underbelly: "You're a sweet flake, Lady. We are scientists. Poetry is for dreamers. You are on a different planet."

Dismissing poetry is dismissing the glory of the imagination. Teaching English to adolescents for twenty years gives me the authority to say, "Kill the imagination and you kill the soul. Kill the soul and you're left with a listless, apathetic creature who can become hopeless or brutal or both. Kill the metaphors and you kill desire; the image magnetizes the movement of the energy."

I'll make this clear as I speak. The tax money that is being withdrawn from arts programs in schools will be spent on prisons. Children have to be educated to hold their passion until their rage, jealousy, lust are transformed by the imagination into poetry, music, art. Otherwise they brutally act out in the streets. The end of culture, the beginning of anarchy. Try to answer a question this way, Marion, instead of putting it in your speech. Otherwise they'll think you're off the track, not talking about healing at all. Remember to explain metaphor as connector between body and soul. Relate this to neuropeptide molecules. Focus on examples.

> The world today hangs by a thin thread, and that is the psyche of man.
>
> —C. G. Jung

I'm going to talk about all of this in Winnipeg. I'm also going to talk about my two analysands who were friends. When Ruth was diagnosed with cancer, she came to me because she had had a dream in which she saw her own tombstone. On it she read, "Beloved daughter of . . . , beloved wife of . . . , beloved mother of. . . ." Her own name and birth and death dates were not there. She herself had not lived. About the same time, Lyn became pregnant. Astonishingly, Ruth began to dream she was pregnant, and Lyn began to have fearsome death dreams. As she realized she was pregnant with herself, Ruth glowed with energy, her radiance increasing as she approached death. Her final dream was of a golden child being born from her crown chakra, gently and relentlessly pushing through the crown of her head. Lyn stayed close to Ruth, even sometimes experienced the darkness of Ruth's tumor growing within herself, a darkness which Ruth did not experience. Lyn saw the Light in the room in which Ruth was dying. She knew Ruth was being initiated into her own wholeness. She also knew such a journey was somewhere in the future for her. That journey began some weeks later, when Lyn gave birth to a stillborn child.

That metaphorical connection between birth and death is very strong in my psyche. All that summer before I was diagnosed I had the inner radiance typical of pregnancy. I was Virgin—one in myself, totally at peace, totally fulfilling my destiny. I remember sitting in the Mennonite rocker in Miranda, rocking, fulfilled. I dreamed about babies—a baby—giving birth to a baby, actually feeling the birth pangs. Here was a new kind of energy—not a baby in a normal, creative way, but another kind of baby whose cells didn't know when to stop growing—went crazy, without pattern. Crazed energy cut off from its desire. A tumor is full of energy encapsulated or not encapsulated. Well, my baby was born by Caesarean section and disposed of—but a baby, nonetheless, that forever changed my life.

October 6, 1994

Winnipeg. Yellow elms embracing avenues. Gracious-ness—wide streets, houses set far back and far apart, with garages, like stables, accessible only from back lanes. Great time with the therapists in the workshop. The unconscious was a basically new world for them. I gave all. Too tired for Grand Rounds. Didn't have the sense of fun, lightness of touch I needed to talk to the medical professionals. Felt the winter storms around me in the late autumn room but said what I wanted to say even if they did think I was naïve. They were polite. I honored their work. I know I wouldn't be here if it weren't for medical expertise. But balance is all! Surely they will recognize there is something more than blood vessels and bone inhabiting a body entrusted to their care. Surely they will know there is something beyond burning, cutting, poisoning in coming to wholeness. Surely they will one day honor subtle body, energy body, light body—by whatever name. Glad to be home.

October 7, 1994

Thinking about passion and the dark feminine and how they are related to creativity and healing. This relationship is one of the biggest tasks of the Crone: holding the opposites in *conscious* aging—holding passion for life in balance with acquiescence in death, holding the spiritual womb always receptive to the creative spirit and choosing the new wholeness born of the new images.

I wasn't able to do that last year. The shocks came and I lost the balance and all faith in any new wholeness. I lost my passion for life—good food, dance, sexuality, music, poetry—all the sensual desires as well as the spiritual. What came to me came; I was grateful. What didn't come didn't; that too was acceptable. The point is there was no passion in either. Nothing could excite me, nothing could hurt me. No "I want." I had transcended everything, including the images that would have opened me to my divinity and my humanity.

I can remember lying in the hospital in Parry Sound with that blissfully unaware diabetic woman for a roommate. She did tests all day with totally crazy results and ate boxes of chocolate cherries her daughter brought her all night. I remember lying in the dim room in the middle of the night watching her silently, systematically licking her lips over one chocolate cherry after another. I remember being startled when I realized I wasn't chuckling over that little morsel of Divine Comedy. I observed everything. I did not participate. And while I looked beatific, I was outside, looking in. That letting go was loss of passion. It was loss of connection to my birthright to life, to my love of luscious, red embodiment. It was my loss of connection to the dark feminine and her lust for life and creativity.

In that disconnecting—I could even say unconscious falling into Death—I lost the sacred connection to my inner masculine. I had no sword at all—nothing that could take hold, discriminate, say, "You are dying, Marion." No differentiation or direction.

The deepest loss of all was loss of my connection to the sacred union within—matter no longer permeated by spirit. I was no longer galvanized by the inner marriage that kept me alive, in life, consciously trying to articulate and write. With that loss of creativity went my power to heal myself. I could not connect with the life force. No energy could get past the darkness in my pelvis to go down into my legs. No life connection to the earth. By the time I began to realize what was happening, even the sexual urge was not strong enough to pull me into life. The passion I associate with the Black Madonna was gone. In her place was the Death Goddess, not in a monstrous form, just seductive, even attractive, luring me into inertia, masked death.

And, of course, her companion was the Demon Lover, that sky energy that lures me off into the heavens under the guise of lover, protector, guide. I was trapped in a false marriage—Death Goddess and Demon Lover—disconnected from my lower chakras and life force. What a fine line! The cul-de-sac in which I have ended so many times in my life! Inertia (looking at the Medusa, petrified, ungrounded) coupled with craving for release into Light—both denial of life. This rung of the spiral is by far the worst. That line between becoming beatific and being lured out of life by the Demon Lover is delicate in me. The secret of staying on

Embodiment: The Virgin *consciously* accepts that she is carrying the Divine Child. Everyday life (matter) is then infused with meaning because it resonates with the symbolic world of the unconscious. Imagination quickens nature.

—MW

Call the world "The vale of Soul-making." . . . Do you not see how necessary a World of Pains and troubles is to school an Intelligence and make it a soul? A Place where the heart must feel and suffer in a thousand diverse ways. Not merely is the Heart a Hornbook, it is the Mind's Bible, it is the Mind's experience.

—*John Keats, Letter to George and Georgiana Keats*

Earth is embodiment. If the Dark Goddess can keep her hold on me through embodiment, I do not fall into the paralysis of her death side, and am therefore not susceptible to the Demon Lover.

Having brought that to consciousness yet again on both the deepest and highest (earth and spirit) levels of the spiral, I see the profound connection between passion, creativity, and healing. Reason and judgment will never again shoot me through the heart. With the "breath, smiles, tears of all my life," I believe consciousness crucial to the survival of the planet. I want to create sacred space open to limitless possibilities for work and research in psyche/soma. I *want* from my survival chakra. My masculinity is now strong enough to protect my feminine values. Thinking of this connection between spirit (Intelligence) and nature (matter), I think of Keats and the heart as hornbook. I love his image of the soul as a little child learning to write, using a very thin piece of horn or bone placed over a beautiful script, learning to write by following the flow of the letters. Thus the child, the soul, eventually finds its own identity through learning by heart.

October 10, 1994

Very quiet Thanksgiving Day. Bruce and Ross and I came to Toronto. Bruce was shocked that Ross and I look forward to our midway snack in McDonald's. We go in there and sink into his McChicken and my McMuffin. There's something so relaxing about sinking, consciously sinking, into the oblivion of McDonald's.

Good to be at the studio again. Snapdragon red sunset.

October 11, 1994

Court. Dread. Need to clarify what is about to happen at ten this morning. Chalmers was so sure everything would go so right! When I agreed to fight for my rights in court over a year ago, I had no idea I'd be so ill, so utterly uninterested in trying to get the money owed to me by the insurance company. Dear God, what is going on? I fight for my life with the medical patriarchs and here I am today fighting with the legal patriarchs. Was it only four days ago I wrote, "My masculinity is now strong enough to protect my feminine values"? Had I been able to retrace my steps last January I would have. But we were already so far into debt in the preliminary hearing, I felt I had to go on to regain our expenses. The company owes me that money; I am going to go into that court this morning and stand to my rights. "Stand to" on one leg. I have to laugh. I, who have talked so much about standpoint, standing on two legs, two feet firmly rooted in the ground, will stand this morning on one leg. I will take Father's heavy cane and go into that court and stand as straight as possible, totally dependent on that piece of wood to hold me up. I will put on my electric blue dress and tell the court I will not accept being cut out of my insurance because the company chose to ignore my phone calls and letters when I attempted to find out my financial status at the time of Fraser's illness. Well, here's looking at you, Kid.

5:00 P.M.

Chalmers picked me up in his vintage Mercedes with its diesel engine. Arrived at Osgoode at 9:00 o'clock. An unknown Toronto opened to me. Splendid architecture, early-twentieth-century broad marble corridors, pillars, wrought-iron gates, exquisite lawns and gardens. Chalmers proudly took me into the inner sanctum in which he was trained. We walked through corridors where one judge after another looked solemnly down on us. The great library was as beautiful as those in Oxford, and the great dome was shining with golden autumn light.

I tried to feel secure in this bastion of justice, but I did not. I did not feel I would walk into a court of law in the next half hour knowing that the law would uphold my rights.

Chalmers went to check location. All the lawyers were running every which way, pulling on their black gowns as they ran through the corridors and up and down the escalators. I was fearful of being knocked over, so I dared to cross this sea of agitated intelligence and stood against the wall. Chalmers joined me. We went to our chamber.

What a morning! I stood in the witness box for almost two hours trying to hear the question exactly and trying to answer it exactly with no extra details at all. "Answer only what you are asked." The cross-examination was very civilly carried out. But I was acutely aware of how deceptive fact can be. No one asked about Fraser's condition physically, or my condition 1991–92. No one noted that he was struggling to accept his death, or that he was in excruciating pain, that he might be thinking about other things far removed from paying an insurance premium. I noted for them the fact that the payments had always been made until the last one. Could they not understand why he missed the payment? I also made clear that they refused to send any documentation to me although I was co-owner of the policy. Why were my requests simply ignored? The insurance company tried to make me look like a dependent woman, dependent on Fraser's decisions, brainless where money was concerned. That was quickly cleared up.

Finally, the judge said it was over and raised the gavel. "I want to say one thing," I said. "Everything looks different in the Presence of Death. Nothing we have said is true so long as we ignore the fact that every detail of these findings was punctuated with excruciating pain." Bang went the gavel. Still, sword did protect soul.

Being in other people's power is a strange experience for me. I can feel them pretending I am not there, nothing in the chair, a sick thing to be overlooked. But then they look into my eyes and fall back, not knowing what to do. They apologize, but do they know for what?

So the case is over for me. It will drag on through more hours for lawyers and dollars.

Slept this afternoon. Spoke to the Writers' Trust tonight. Terribly nervous. Theater at Trinity College filled to capacity. Couldn't quite get there. Stood up, light came on. I could see Edith and Rita in the seats in front of me and Chalmers to the side, Ross and Bruce in the back. My ego surrendered and gradually I felt the dance between me and the audience begin. Loved them, they loved me and the humor danced. That magical spirit was present. Lively reception afterward in Massey Hall.

October 12–13, 1994

Stayed in Toronto. Working with some of my analysands still moving toward closure of their analysis. If they do the ritual preparation, go back through their journals, and recognize who they were at the beginning of the analysis, what their prime symbols are, how they and their symbols have transformed in the process, who they are now—if they allow that to come to consciousness, then they can sacrifice the analytic container and be free. They can claim the no longer projected energy as their own and recognize their real parents in God and Sophia, however they wish to name them. They can take responsibility for their own maturity. Together we can close the analytic container and release our energies in new directions.

I have to do my work in relationship to all of this with each of them. I too need to be released. It will take some months. That's fine. I can see in their psyches the rupture that my sudden disappearance caused last November. For several of them, that was a repetition of the primal rupture from their birth mother. If we're careful, we can redeem both the original trauma and the repetition. We'll move at each individual pace.

October 14, 1994

Ross wheeled me around the Barnes Exhibition at the AGO. Dear man! His sensation function is being forced to work overtime these days. He'd be so intent on the next picture that he'd bump the chair into people. They'd look at me as if I'd hit them. When he'd push the chair to the spot where he could see a painting, I would find myself eye to eye with some forgotten little animal or a lost rose or carpet design—the nether regions of these familiar works of art, regions that I had never seen before. Very interesting, occasionally funny, sometimes tragic—details that were often contrapuntal to the upper parts of the picture. In spite of the static, we did see the light emanating from these splendid impressionists' paintings. Forerunners of Einstein's $E=mc^2$.

Feel great intimacy with children in go-carts. They look at me as if I'm a big kid. They aren't sure whether to trust me or not. I seem to be one with them, but not quite, because my go-cart is much bigger than theirs. I guess second childhood is like this. But damn it, I'm not ready to accept a wheelchair yet—people bending over and kissing "poor Marion."

Did you come of your own free will or did you come by compulsion?

—*Baba Yaga*

October 15, 1994

Returned to Sydenham from Toronto. Felt very sad saying good-bye to Bruce. Feel the precariousness of our good-byes with this disease lurking in the background. So does he. Cannot forget looking into Fraser's frightened eyes on Jan. 15, 1992 and knowing he was dying, and knowing that he knew. It was our last good-bye in this dimension. The rest was transitional space and death.

October 16, 1994

Incredible autumn! Try to walk to the park every day to Jack and Olga's trees. Recite poems to try to keep a steady pace.

Season of mists and mellow fruitfulness,
  Close bosom-friend of the maturing sun;
Conspiring with him how to load and bless
  With fruit the vines that round the thatch-
    eaves run. . . .

(*John Keats, "To Autumn"*)

October 17, 1994

Went to Dr. Cohen. She says the results show severe osteoporosis and severe osteoarthritis in my lower back and fifth lumbar vertebra, exacerbated by radiation. Well, when I was in England last year, I went from not walking to being able to move quite well.

Dear Sophia, let me not lose hope.

October 18, 1994

Phoned the clinic to see what Dr. Thomas made of the scans. Have an appointment for his clinic on Friday. People say, "It must be terrible waiting for the results." I don't find it so. Until I'm told I have cancer, I don't worry. I feel I'm on borrowed time, loving every walk through this season of gold and burnished blue. Never was such an autumn in London's recorded history. Day after day, warm as summer, and flowers not bitten by frost.

An epiphany in the garden this afternoon. I was cleaning the birdbath. As I turned to pour fresh water, brilliant sunlight caught the one stray sunflower. There, eighteen inches from my face, was a golden mandala. Perfect petals surrounding rows of nut-brown seeds in perfect symmetry. Matter magnifying spirit. I felt god and goddess in the ecstasy of love right there in our little garden. The conception of spirit so exquisitely made manifest in form. Sunflowers, like heliotropes, love to turn their faces toward the sun to drink in the golden elixir. Thank you, Sophia, for your message so eloquently delivered.

October 19, 1994

Decided to do yoga with Judith [friend]. She knows what she's doing and doesn't push me beyond where my back is able to go. Her big yoga bolster is the most comforting thing I've had. It opens my back when I put it exactly under my knees, opens my whole torso, and I sleep like a baby. Her exercises release the spasm that cuts off my leg.

For the divine sparks of autumn, thank you, Sophia. Now that I'm better I feel the strength of my bond to you even deeper because I feel I'm on my own now. I feel others' prayers supporting me, but the crisis is over.

> The divine sparks of the Universe are one in Sophia. As Bride, she unites with Bridegroom in the unified Godhead.
>
> —MW

The adrenaline isn't firing my body as it used to. We've settled into normal living. I'm realizing that I had to give up my practice. Who am I without my work? Here I am back in the little pastoral city where I was born, graduated from college, married, taught school for twenty-one years—and left. How do I reconnect? Do I reconnect?

October 21, 1994

Ross and I went to the clinic this morning. I like it—lovely paintings, strong upholstered chairs, good colors—olive green, dark rose—and exquisite tropical fish in three large aquariums. So peaceful to enjoy a hot cup of coffee and a quarter doughnut and dream with the grace of the fish. Actually thought of setting up my big aquarium again, but decided I couldn't handle the cleaning of it without the strength in my back. So I enjoy them in the big waiting room.

Dr. Thomas wasn't there. I talked to the nurse, who is her cheerful, chattering self. Yes, I am holding my weight. No more blood. Yes, I'm eating the yellowest and greenest vegetables—ten half-cup servings every day—not too good with the raw yet—but yes, squash, pumpkin, yams, carrots, and broccoli. I feel yellow and green. Yes, eight glasses of my special water every day and up four times every night. Pain anywhere? My back and legs. Dr. MacNeil will come to see me.

Dr. MacNeil, a quiet, unprepossessing man, comes in. He says he read the scan with the other doctors. They agree it is metastasized bone cancer on the inside of my sacrum. He shoots me through my heart close range. I just keep looking at him. No voice to respond.

"I'm sorry if I've spoiled your weekend," he says.

Go out to Ross reading his newspaper in the waiting room. He takes one look at my face and knows there must be a cancer diagnosis. My voice is very low. He receives

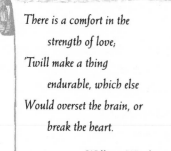

There is a comfort in the strength of love;
'Twill make a thing endurable, which else
Would overset the brain, or break the heart.

—*William Wordsworth,*
"Michael"

the news quietly. We sit and hold each other's hand. A lady our age begins to cry across the coffee table. "She's been here," I think, looking at her thin, drawn face. Her husband too begins to cry. None of us speaks. We sit stone still. We've known each other forever. Eventually Ross says, "Well, darling," and we stand up and drive to Sydenham in silence.

Dear Sophia—be around and within me—my circle of light in the darkness. Break my heart open to a richer understanding of Incarnation. I feel my suffering flesh, I feel my darkness. If it is my time, I'm ready. But I do not feel death in my bones in spite of what the doctor says. Oh, come into my darkness, light every cell of my body with your love. Light of your light, light of your darkness—dearly Beloved, let your moonlight shine in me. In this Harrowing of Hell, hold your daughter close. Here is the final unveiling. In the dark night ahead, give me the strength to bring forth a new baby. In the fullness of time, let the child live in my womb, my new spiritual womb. May we live Incarnation.

October 22—23, 1994

Very still day. Autumn burgundies and dark blues. Canada geese and mallard ducks playing in the sunbeams. That stillness of autumn that revels in its own beauty before the deathblow strikes.

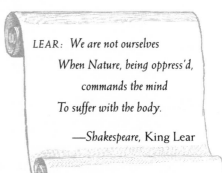

LEAR: *We are not ourselves*
When Nature, being oppress'd,
commands the mind
To suffer with the body.

—Shakespeare, King Lear

An adorable skunk wandered into Bob's garden today. A sheer glory of black and white with a Cyrano de Bergerac plume of a tail. Bob's squirrel cage was still there and somehow this dear visitor got into it. No fuss. No bother. She sensed she was trapped. She went all around the four sides, putting her little white paw out as far as she could. She explored every possibility of escape, and then, knowing she could not, instead of running like a mad squirrel around the cage until she collapsed, she lay down in the warm sun and went to sleep. When the trapper came, she didn't spray. He shot her with a drug pellet and took her away. But what a regal coming together of opposites—what dignity!

October 24, 1994

I am going to the clinic, yet again, to find out whether I have cancer in my spine. I won't believe it until I talk to Dr. Thomas. This is a momentous day—one of the before-and-after days of a lifetime. I am very aware—Ross is very aware. We are very close. Bruce and Cherry and Luke are close by their phones. So are Marion, Elinor, and Jill.

Dear God, give me the strength to deal with this creatively. I feel doom lower if he says "Yes, metastasized cancer." I can't fight against that. I can, however, still keep working with food, exercise, visualization to try to live as fully as I can. Please, if it be Thy will, give me time to write the book, my life book on the Demon Lover. Yes, please let this be the ultimate scare. I have felt it in my marrow. I don't need further fear. I pray for direction. Bone cancer is very different from endometrial cancer.

Phoned the clinic. No response from Dr. Thomas. Putting one foot ahead of the other, concentrating on preparing vegetables, and doing visualization on my back. My celadon green covering for my single bed/sofa arrived today. The last piece finally in place. Diane's stained glass creates breathtaking blues and mauves on the soft carpet, and the greens with the terra-cotta walls are warm and sensuous. All my office furniture from Toronto is now integrated except I need two small pillows of the water lily pattern to integrate the couches. I took the arm covers apart. That's just enough material for Doris to make the pillows. Dear Doris, how beloved you are! How faithfully you have fielded calls and kept me in touch.

Strange how I can care so much about the details of this house knowing the death sentence is in the wings. Compensation, no doubt! If I'm concentrating on the exact shade of green and how the sun falls through the unicorn in my window, I don't worry about death. Light permeating matter. Like Notre Dame in Paris. That's where I first realized the medieval love of glass came from its sense of the cathedral as matter mother. The spirit light permeated the magnificent matter of the windows and the whole body of the cathedral. "Permeable" is a big word in my psyche right now.

October 25, 1994

Waited all day for the call. Did interview with Pythia. Waited until 4:00 P.M. Phoned Dr. Thomas to find out when I should go to see him. Finally reached him. "Come tomorrow morning for a biopsy—eighty-thirty A.M.," he said. Still hope!

October 26, 1994

7:55 A.M.

Phoned clinic to find out where to go. Got Dr. Thomas. "Phone the clinic desk," he said.

I did.

"Don't come," the receptionist said. "Biopsy canceled."

"I just spoke to Dr. Thomas," I said.

"Canceled," she said.

Phoned his nurse instantly.

"Canceled," she said.

"May I speak to him?" I said.

"Gone," she said. "I'll tell him to phone when he can."

Sat most of the day in the wing chair tracing the yellow pattern with my finger. Why canceled? No hope?

3:00 P.M.

Message from his nurse. Dr. Mosher, the head, and Dr. Thomas had a meeting to look at the scan. Because the tumor is located on the inside of the sacrum, a biopsy is impossible. Too dangerous for the legs. Too many nerves.

4:30 P.M.

Talking on red phone in kitchen. Dr. Thomas says, "No point in biopsy. It is cancer—metastasized cancer. Too dangerous to try to biopsy."

"Prognosis?" I ask.

"Bad," he says. "Very bad."

"How long?" I ask.

"Two months to two years. Less rather than more."

I can't move from the kitchen counter. Can't step, can't hold on to a chair. Catatonic. Ross comes to the kitchen. Puts me down on a chair. He makes tea.

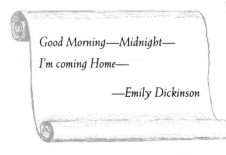

Good Morning—Midnight—
I'm coming Home—

—Emily Dickinson

October 27, 1994

Didn't tell my two analysands this morning anything. No tears. No desire. No yellow and green vegetables. No meditation. Just a walk to see the last fires of the trees. Ross asked Martin and Ann to come over. Dear souls, they came, very quietly. Here's Martin walking around life and instant death with his heart condition. As a medical doctor he carries authority for me and for Ross. He brought champagne. Exactly right! What were we celebrating? Death? Life? Life-in-Death? None of us knew, but I desired that champagne and we all drank to the last drop. Put Barbra Streisand's new CD on the player.

Martin said, "Do what you want to do, Marion. Live, really live—go around the world, buy clothes, anything. Do it."

I didn't have to think one thought about what I would do to really live.

"I have no desire to go around the world again," I said. "I've lived it. I've loved it. No clothes. No. I want to stay—I desire—I choose to stay right here in my beautiful home, to concentrate on my preparations for the transition—and to write. No conflict."

Martin and Ann found that strange. But here in my space my whole realm is present. Dearest Ross, my dearest family and friends present in body or spirit,

Her *lips* were red, her *looks* were
   free,
Her *locks* were *yellow as gold:*
Her *skin* was *white as leprosy,*
The *Nightmare* LIFE-IN-DEATH *was*
   she,
Who thicks man's blood with cold.

   —*Samuel Taylor Coleridge,*
   "The Rime of the Ancient
   Mariner"

Our revels now are ended.

—*Shakespeare,* The Tempest

my books at my fingertips, my pen, my paper, my tape deck, my trees, my geese, my ducks—everything—and space to pray and dance as I can. Dear Sophia, thank you. I have lived and therefore I can die. Give me strength to hold my eyes open, steadfastness to reject sentimentality. Pour your love over Ross, our family, and friends.

October 28, 1994—Friday

Nothing—never—lay in the dark last night, still inside, still outside. "This is what it's going to be like underground," I thought.

Felt the oppression of weight on top of me. It was only darkness, but it took my breath away.

October 29, 1994—Saturday

Autumn stillness—inner stillness.

What is ceasing to exist? My body going back to dust. Earth to earth, dust to dust, ashes to ashes. I touch my warm skin and try to imagine it cold. Think of our compost heap in which earth does go back to earth. This is not metaphor. So be it. My soul will be free.

The trees are too bronze, too burgundy, too exquisite against the burnished sky. I walk through the wind and weep for their beauty.

She sees a candle lit on the window sill of the hospital room and finds that the candle suddenly goes out. Fear and anxiety ensue as the darkness envelops her. Suddenly, the candle lights on the other side of the window and she awakens.

—*Marie-Louise von Franz,
on Dreams & Death*

Ross and I went to the Wonderland nursery today. Bought yew bushes to create a box hedge in our garden. The calendulas are still singing.

October 30, 1994—Sunday

Took communion this morning at 8:00 o'clock mass. Experienced myself on the other side of the veil looking at my dying self kneeling at the altar. Felt released. Free of this vale of tears.

Canceled ticket to San Diego. Very difficult to accept my failure to live up to my responsibilities.

Dearest Sophia, thank you for giving me time to experience this autumn and strength to take it in. Still roses in the garden.

October 31, 1994

Dr. Thomas phoned. "I've ordered an MRI to be done at University Hospital on Monday, November 14. Since we can't see this tumor, and can't biopsy it, we will do a magnetic resonance imaging scan." My doctor is still trying. Apparently a strong magnetic field is used to generate signals from atoms in the body. A computer then converts these signals into a picture that will show the exact location of the tumor and something of its nature.

Dr. Thomas said it wouldn't hurt to fly to New York. Dr. Cohen signed my insurance claim

Hope springs eternal in the human breast.

—*Alexander Pope, "An Essay on Man"*

form to change my ticket. I saw what she put on the medical sheet—metastasized bone cancer. Something in me screamed "NO," and fell in a heap. Said nothing.

November 2, 1994 — Wednesday

Ross and I flew to La Guardia, New York. Dear God, the memories—Marjory, Gramercy Park, our honeymoon and running barefoot through the street cleaners' hose after dancing till dawn in the Stork Club, chaperoning the South students, and skipping through Central Park, ballets, art galleries, concerts, New Year's Eve at Lincoln Center.

Yes, and Wayne and Mary Clare coming to meet us after their wedding to share a toast on the *Queen Elizabeth* before Shelley, Ross, and I set off for our sabbatical in England—the anticipation of our year in London matched by the anticipation of their first year together. The sun was hot on the deck as we laughed our way through champagne and strawberries. Looking back, I think there was more fear than hope in our gaiety—a detachment, a letting go from land—in all of us.

And yes, I remember the coming home in '71—Ross and I up at cold dawn to commune with the Hudson and America in an effort to make a psychic return to this side of the Atlantic. We were both anxious, pacing the deck. We were off the boat early and drove into Manhattan to have lunch at Sardi's before we drove to London. We did make rituals of passage to bring our journeys to consciousness. We never slept our way through. I won't sleep my way through this one either. Though this is a sea with a difference.

Have a generous suite in the Beekman Tower Hotel near the United Nations Building. Never lived in this part

of New York before. It's good because I can cook what we can eat.
Restaurants are still impossible.

Saw *Three Tall Women*. Great.
Three phases of womanhood, each
wearing different phases of pearls,
different but similar hairdos—
Mother, Virgin, Crone, each looking
at her own phase from a different
vantage point. I have those vantage
points in my journals. Try, Bubbles.

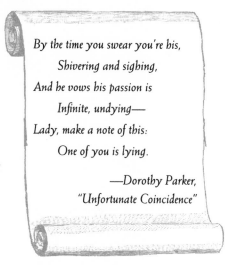

By the time you swear you're his,
Shivering and sighing,
And he vows his passion is
Infinite, undying—
Lady, make a note of this:
One of you is lying.

—Dorothy Parker,
"Unfortunate Coincidence"

November 3, 1994

We went to the United Nations Building, through secu-
rity, into the dining room overlooking the river. Between
the main course and dessert, Open Center honored me
with an award for my contribution to the feminine in the
twentieth century. I was very quiet as I gave my response.
Robert Bly also received an award for his contribution to
men and poetry. Yes, it was worth making the effort to
come to New York—a summing-up of my life, a recognition, a joyous receiving by my friends, Adele and Ilana, and
so many young people. There was a completion and somehow it was right in New York. This city has been a catalyst
in our marriage, and a focal point for my work all over
America.

November 4, 1994

Ross and I walked in Central Park, went to the Met.
Neither of us mentions that we will probably never walk

here hand in hand again. But that knowledge enhances every moment. We are alive to everything.

November 7–8, 1994

Exhaustion. Couldn't wake out of the depths. Stayed in Toronto to rest before driving home. Jill phoned from Palo Alto, sensed there was something wrong. I told her, heard my own flat voice, could feel myself vacating this body. With strangers, I can act. With her, I cannot. She was silent. We hung up.

Later she phoned again. "Marion, why don't you get a second opinion? You don't need to accept this diagnosis as absolute. I have a friend in the radiology department at Stanford. Let me talk to him."

Some light went on in our conversation. Some spark was ignited. Something screamed, "Yes," and fell silent— one crack of lightning bolting through a jet-black night.

"OK, Jill," I said, but I didn't dare hope. I was thankful for a voice outside the darkness strong enough, kind enough, to reach my soul. Talking with a consciousness outside made me realize the depth of my despair. I feel my medical doctors have almost given up hope. That note from Dr. Cohen I happened to see on my cancellation insurance felt like a deathblow. I told her I did not believe I am dying. She thinks I am in denial—a natural phase after a death sentence.

November 9, 1994

Jill phoned. She had received the letter I wrote after the red phone call of October 26. Had talked to her friend Dr.

Mindelzun. He said he would be happy to talk to me. Meantime I galvanized myself to phone Dr. Alastair Cunningham at Princess Margaret, made appointment for Friday, 25th. Feel tiny gusts of hope, but not daring to pray for wind.

Tonight phoned Dr. Bob Mindelzun. He was kind, assertive, treated me as if I were alive and worth talking to. He asked me questions that I should have had answers to, but I never thought to ask them.

1. Exactly what am I being treated for?
2. Is the problem located in one place?
3. Where am I being treated—in what part of my body exactly?
4. How do I know this is a tumor?
5. Who is the captain of the ship? Which doctor knows everything that is going on?
6. How advanced is this tumor? Is it a primary tumor?

He suggested I find an internist or gynecologist who is captain of the ship—one person who knows me and all about my treatments. That doctor may send me to a specialist, but he/she has to have all the facts and know all the treatments. Rarely is radiation done without a biopsy. Need to know 100 percent before going into radiation again. The radiation specialist has to know for sure what he is radiating and where.

He echoed my fear of accepting radiation again. I think it would destroy any bones I have left. I told him about my twelve-year problem with my back and how this pain is exactly in the same place, acting the same way, and how I finally was able to walk last year before the cancer. Told him of the family problem in that area.

Dr. Mindelzun asked me to send copy of CAT scan.

Hung up the phone. I felt genuinely respected in my personhood and breath came into my lower rib cage for the first time in weeks. Dr. Mindelzun said he would take primary responsibility for looking into my case, consult with a group of experts from the tumor board at Stanford, review all the findings, and make a joint recommendation.

November 10, 1994

Ross and I drove home to London through the soft autumn mists and dark green autumn wheat. Music on the car radio for Remembrance Day, November 11. Memories of that anguished ride through Alsace-Lorraine with miles and miles and miles of simple crosses. Thousands upon thousands of young men, food for fodder. They never had their lives. What's all the fuss about, Marion? You're 66, one little life.

> *They shall grow not old, as we that are left grow old:*
> *Age shall not weary them, nor the years condemn.*
> *At the going down of the sun and in the morning*
> *We will remember them.*
>
> *(Laurence Binyon, "For the Fallen")*

Do we? Do we take responsibility for the freedom they died for?

November 11, 1994

Ross and I went to Mt. Pleasant Cemetery to buy a plot today. We hated the whole business, but I'm trying to get the wills in order, buy membership in the Memorial Society, and buy the plot. The receptionist showed us a place right beside a water faucet. I didn't think much of that. Didn't fancy being wet and cold throughout eternity. Besides, it was the middle of a row. Suddenly feared being claustrophobic. I never sit anywhere but on the end of an aisle if I can help it. We

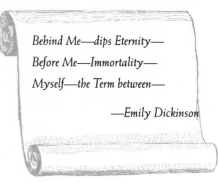

Behind Me—dips Eternity—
Before Me—Immortality—
Myself—the Term between—

—Emily Dickinson

confused realities! What possible difference does it make? Tearful Beckett laughter.

Many families with flowers at the veterans' plots today. We stood a long time honoring and remembering, especially the ones we loved who never came back. How their wives and sweethearts and mothers were undone by their going! One generation, in fact two generations of the finest manhood their countries had to offer wiped out. The speed with which our social order is collapsing had its roots in those two wars.

Having been an air force officer, Ross wanted to be buried near the veterans. He felt at home there. So we put our check down for $1400. Paid our respects to Mother and Father in Mt. Pleasant and to my grandmother and grandfather. Seems strange to be the next in line. Our visitation was a little too intimate today.

Driving home, Ross said, "As a Baha'i I can't be buried more than three hours from where I die. I don't intend to stay in London for fear I might die too far away to be buried in that plot." When we got home, I phoned to ask the woman to return the check.

November 12, 1994

Still vigilant: ten servings of green and yellow vegetables, eight glasses of water, a walk, several visualizations.

I look in the mirror—my eyes seem brighter, my skin clearer, my body stronger. Maybe it is denial, but it doesn't feel so. Still, I have to admit I have lost 3½ inches in height and my skeletal frame is shrinking. I may yet die the petite person I once yearned to be.

November 14, 1994

MRI this morning. Coffin experience. The narrow bed rolls into a long, dark tube. The door closes, my face a few inches from the cylinder. I lie flat and still. Start to cough; can't raise my hands to my face; can't cough deeply, can't stop coughing, afraid I'll mess up the whole thing and not have any results until another test after Christmas.

Magnetic resonance imaging! A knocking noise starts—1, 2, 3, 4—like an ax striking an old tree in a closed barn. Quite regular—thud, thud, thud, thud. Then a light, dancing rhythm begins, like children dancing in little clogs. Then a very serious rumbling indeed. "It's imaging the tumor," I think. "It's big; it's full; it's heavy; it's black." Rumbling resonates through my bones. I try to stop choking. More knocking, more dancing, more foreboding rumbles. Then it is over. Not bad at all!

Went to Victoria/Westminster Hospital this afternoon, straight to the library and asked for copies of my scans. Jill says these belong to me, so I had no hesitation in asking for them. I received the whole bundle. Didn't see any doctor I knew. I'll take these to Dr. Cunningham.

November 15, 1994

Drove to Toronto, immediately to Dr. Cunningham. After all my daring in getting a second opinion, getting the bundle and finding him—he wasn't a medical doctor. "I'm sorry to disappoint you," he said. He was so kind I didn't care. He's a psychologist who counsels cancer patients. He assisted the healing process of his own cancer with spiritual work and lifestyle changes. We had a splendid interview. He referred me to Dr. Fyles at Princess Margaret, so he will give the official second opinion. Still, I trust Dr. Mindelzun, so I bundled the bundle up and sent it priority post to California. I don't mean to deceive anyone, but I have to do something to save myself. Good fox, Marion.

November 16, 1994

Had to rush back from Toronto for an early appointment with Dr. Thomas. Arrived at the clinic. He wasn't there. I couldn't believe it. Why did he order this MRI if he thinks it's over?

Ross and I sat down to gather ourselves.

The woman at the desk called me over. "Why are you here?" she asked.

"To see Dr. Thomas," I said.

"He's in the simulator," she said.

I heard "incinerator." I had told him I could not take any more radiation. "You will crawl," he said, "when the pain is bad enough." So here he was encouraging the stenciling in preparation for palliative radiation. However, I did hobble down to see him. He looked desperate, straight into my eyes. He put his hand full on my back.

"I know it is terrible," he whispered.

He *meant* it. Maybe all our misses reflect his caring too much. Certainly, his gesture was spontaneous. I silently honored his recognition of feeling. He convinced me to have the stenciling so we'd be ready when the pain came. I lay down. The smiling technician babbled, "How are you today?"

"TERRIBLE," I bellowed from the table.

November 17, 1994

Walk with Mary every Thursday afternoon. Still golden warm autumn. Sophia permeates everything—light bouncing off the river, splashing through the ducks, radiant in the tracery of the white birch against the azure blue sky. Mary and I strode with Her in our bones, breathing deep into our bellies, opening our arms wide to receive Her.

Had appointment with Needham Funeral Home to join Memorial Society. They had to cancel. Why do all my efforts to get this death ritual together fail? Wrong time, I hope.

November 18, 1994

Bal and Chandra here for tea. Chandra on her way to India for a year—not sure she'll ever see me again. Strange distancing with everyone. They are in one living room; I am in another. Having tea, enjoying cheesecake and cherry topping is part of life to them. Tea and cheesecake don't belong to my reality anymore. I can hardly drink or eat or converse. I am transported onto some other plane. I'm looking at the world from a spaceship, even looking at the clinic from a spaceship.

Don't belong anywhere. Have to remember to breathe, especially at night. Ross is so precious. My heart breaks for him. I look at his white hair and frail body and wonder what will happen when he knows he is forever alone. The ways he touches me now, puts his arm around me in sleep, I know he is thinking of the times when he will reach out and I will not be there. And I think, "Where in God will I be?" Life after death used to be thinkable. Now my imagination can't get beyond the moment of death—not even that far.

November 21, 1994

Talked to Dr. Bob tonight about my scans. Was shaking so much I could barely hold the phone. He sensed my terror.

"I think I may be bringing some hope," he began. Then I could hear him. "There are a lot of arthritic changes in your spine," he said. I write everything down because in my nervousness I can't remember, but I can hear and write without my brain taking it in, then I can study it afterward.

"Osteoporosis and osteoarthritis certainly. There is a fluid collection, but I do not believe it is a malignant process. Difficult making a definite diagnosis with this scan," he said. "Go to a major center if necessary—Toronto, Mayo Clinic, Massachusetts General—find out what it is before you have more radiation. More radiation may exacerbate the condition. Get a gynecologist and an oncologist. Review findings. Find out what needs to be treated."

Felt his energy opening mine. Toronto feels right.

"If the prognosis is bad," he said, "will the irradiation improve it? Is the treatment palliative or curative? In that area, will it hurt the other organs? Is there a problem in other areas of the body? Any vital organs? Be demanding."

He distinguished between an oncologist and a radiation therapist. An oncologist is an internist who has taken specialized training in tumors. He will make decisions and independent evaluations, but may send a patient to a radiation therapist. He himself usually uses chemotherapy. A radiation therapist is trained in tumors, usually only malignant tumors.

So energized after this conversation and telling it to Ross. Glimmerings of a New Day.

November 22, 1994

Ross came with me to Princess Margaret. I need him with me. And he now wants to come. He needs to meet the doctor. Met Dr. Fyles late this afternoon. He was kind, good at making a relationship, thorough in his examination. Unfortunately he didn't have the scans back from California. They must have been trapped in customs. So I have to wait for him to see them.

He isn't satisfied with the MRI from London, so the next one is set for December 9 at Princess Margaret. Then we'll wait again to find out if it's "the big C" or not. Truth is I don't mind waiting. That "believing" it was cancer was so terrible, so black, so disorienting that I'd rather be in this limbo with not much hope, but a little. I can stay with my disciplines more easily when I hope for life. I would use very different disciplines if I believed I was dying.

November 23, 1994

Saw a few analysands today. Good to be in normal routine again. I'm asking them to take time to reflect on who they were when they came into analysis, then to follow the natural gradient of their energy, see where it took them, what it brought to consciousness, where they are now and what they have within themselves to carry their soul to wherever she needs to BE. I ask them to figure out what their sacrifice is (the fatted calf, not the scrawny one), what food is important in their ritual (if there is food) and to bring these and anything else they choose to make this ritual totally their own. It may take a year for some of them to reach this place, but there is no hurry in Sophia's time. In closing the analytic container, we are opening each other to possible metamorphosis. So often I wish they could act on the immense shifts of perception the dreams are bringing. So often I want to say, "You're talking like a caterpillar. Can't you feel your great yellow wings?" But I cannot push them. I have to concentrate until their images ignite their energy. No rush, no push, no pull.

November 24–25, 1994

More work with analysands. Quite enjoying being in Toronto, enjoy aloneness of letting my soul soar on its own to unknown places. Working hard every day on visualization. So far the pain is not nearly so bad as before I began this hourly meditation. I do it whenever I feel like it, walking, sitting, resting. Judith sent me a painting of the sacrum which I framed in order to look at it any time I wish. It shows the entire pelvic cradle in red, orange, and yellow colors so I can feel golden light coming from and going into my pelvic bone structure. I put my own hot hands on it to direct the energy more strongly. I'm trying to get the sense of that pelvic bowl which roots and supports the spine, trying to find the sense of equanimity there that can balance my whole body. In the middle of the night, I pour energy into my sacrum and try to listen to the tumor that is lodged in front of it. I feel the vertebrae opening when I breathe into them, feel more relaxed and full of sleep. How exhausted my body must have been!

As I think of this golden bowl supporting the fierce spiritual energy descending, attracted to matter, and Earth energy equally fierce ascending, attracted to spirit, I feel the inner marriage yearning to be consummated right there within me.

I feel the power of this imagery because it is the conflict of my life—matter energy rising up into spirit until it becomes ungrounded and spirit energy thrusting down through shoulders and trunk yearning to permeate pelvis and legs, yet terrified of losing its wings. I have never held that balance except in dance. I find it there because I become music; my body finds its balance and I can dance hour after hour without rest. This new

---

The Latin word *sacer* means both "holy" and "cursed." It is the ancestor of familiar English words like "sacred" and "sacrifice," as well as of the name of a small triangular bone that forms both the back of the pelvis and the base of the spine. Known to anatomists as the *os sacrum*, literally the "holy bone," it was given this appellation, according to one legend, because it was believed to be eternal and so the "seat" of the body's resurrection.

—Richard Rosen,
"The Holy Bone," Yoga Journal

death threat releases the arrow that hits the bull's-eye of this conflict.

Moreover, it brings back my archetypal snake dream. A voice told me my hymns could not reach heaven and I would never place the bouquet of red and white roses in the cross at the center of the temple until the mess was cleaned up in my basement. When I picked my way down an old moss-covered spiral staircase I had not known existed, I saw an immense black snake frenetically trying to connect its head to an ominously still wheel of life. It knew the water that had now become a stagnant lagoon should be carried up on the wheel to become the fresh water of life. So long as the snake (life force) couldn't connect to the wheel, my body was drowning in edema. The Presence who was with me in the dream stayed with me in my visualizations and body work. Together, months later, we finally helped the snake to connect to the wheel, and to push down on the spokes with its head and thus keep the wheel of life turning. The stagnant pool on my body transformed into living water without dialysis. The kidney problem was thus resolved twenty years ago. Now it is a bone problem or maybe cancer—a tumor holding powerful energy that needs to be re-created and released to allow energy to flow up and down. Physically in my body, the sacred bone

The muladhara [first chakra] is the starting point and foundation of our spiritual quest. . . . The sacrum is the "earth" that supports the spine. . . . If the sacrum is properly positioned, these two forces—which represent the complementary human aspirations of descent into matter and ascent toward spirit—course smoothly through the spine, and we live a fully supported existence.

—November–December 1993,
Yoga Journal

is the site of the inner marriage. Is lower back pain a symptom crying out for balance between spirit and matter?

The other thing that's so interesting in the painting is the key at the bottom of the sacrum. I remember seeing my Celtic cross in a dream. At a distance, it looked like a key, but as I came closer, it was my cross in leaping flames and the voice said, "Your key is your cross." Again, the holding of the opposites between earth and spirit. Considering my Celtic cross has always looked like my feminine body to me, my body itself is burning in the fire of passion, physical and spiritual.

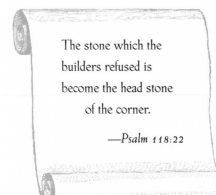

Burn off my rust and my deformity,
Restore Thine image so much,
by Thy grace,
That Thou may'st know me,
and I'll turn my face.

—John Donne,
"Good Friday, 1613,
Riding Westward"

That's where the issue is won or lost.

I love the flowers at the bottom with the long stems moving through holes in the sacrum. I can feel those flowers in my feet and visualize the energy moving through my sacrum, down my legs, into my toes.

Cancer: what is it now to me? It has to do with bringing to consciousness all that I once simply accepted as part of my life. I took my body for granted. I took Nature for granted. Although I was always aware of natural beauty, I didn't feel it inside as I do now. I didn't experience it as Sophia, as God made manifest, as immanent light, light permeating matter. I didn't experience it as sacred. Certainly, I never took my sacrum seriously. Now I see it as pivotal to my healing.

The stone which the builders refused is become the head stone of the corner.

—Psalm 118:22

What is very clear to me now is that the Black Madonna, who has been so dear to me ever since India, is in fact Nature herself. She is black, luscious, nurturing, cherishing. She is the life force—even as a tiny aster breaking through rock is the life force—perseverance and strength and passion. She is in my body. Dare I say, "She is my body"? I have worshiped her in Nature with increasing awe all my life, but the stone I rejected was also Her, my body. So long as that stone is rejected, it remains stone, can become a hard tumor in the sacrum, encapsulated as a time bomb. If that rejected stone is loved, is recognized as sacred—the cross, the key, the fire—the energy is released, the light flows through the darkness—as the light shines through the black sapphire in my grandmother's brooch. If I can release that rejected stone into energy flowing through my body, it becomes the cornerstone, incarnate, the feminine energy of God, the serpent energy no longer cursed but blessed.

November 26, 1994

Going through a convulsion. Feel as though the past is past, the future I don't know, the ground I'm walking on is not secure. Can feel my legs actually pulling up when I try to put them on the ground. They have no alternative but to go onto the ground, but my toes are curled, I'm toeing in, my shins hurt, my knees are fire. Shades of my doctor telling me I'd be in a walker by Christmas. Everything in me said, "No. No way." But what is going on? I can feel my hip sockets rotating as I try to step ahead. My leg swings out in a circle on its own before it lands. Very awkward. Convulsive fear when I go out. Do my legs not want to go any further? I keep talking to them, letting them talk to me. They're afraid; they don't want to stay if all that lies ahead is pain. They don't want to be grounded anymore— not even in the park. I tell them, "Don't give up. I know, I'm afraid too. We'll have to put up with this fear for a while yet."

When I let them talk, they do relax. I gave them a long footbath in Dr. Heimer's twelve mineral salts tonight. Then did reflexology with goat's milk cream. They purred and stopped jumping around. I think they need extra attention.

Last week I admit I lost my disciplines. I did not stay with my green and yellow vegetables. I did not walk every day. I did not meditate every day. On the deepest level, I gave up. Pull up your socks, Bubbles. Let's stay with it. Face the reality, accept your vulnerability and keep walking.

Celebrated Tom's sixtieth birthday tonight, rather than the 28th. Tom was fabulous—full of love and tears. So different from the ordered, restrained man he used to be. Lovely with Adam, Dory, and Marion. As we were making our tributes, I was too shy to read my letter to him, but afterward I thought, "Dear God, if I can't read in front of these dear friends, what has become of me?" Ten minutes after saying, "No," I humbled myself by saying, "Yes." I had to honor forty years of friendship. I know I'm not present. This repeated stepping back alarms me—this detached looking on. Still, this detachment is not indifference. I think it may be the root of pure love—love with no strings attached.

November 27, 1994

Wrote Ross's 72nd birthday poem, signed it Lady Lazarus. Made his favorite cordon bleu chicken and sugarless date dessert. We celebrated tonight. Drank a grape juice toast to William Blake on his birthday. Then to Ross. So glad we had that sparkling party for him two years ago. Will never forget him looking at the seventy full-blown white roses and seventy white burning tapers and the Sacher torte he could only taste. I guess I shouldn't have made it for the thirty-six birthdays when he still adored chocolate with a soupçon of apricot. Too much sugar. No, Marion, stop it. You can't think that way. You've tried to live as consciously as you could at each phase of the journey.

November 28, 1994

To Toronto. Important session with Helga. She opened up my back as I cannot. She listened to my story calmly, but I couldn't look into her eyes as I told it. Very unusual. She made notes. Are we avoiding the depth of the intimacy?

November 29–30, 1994

More ritual closures with analysands. So powerful! All honoring with everything within them the process we have been through, and now taking their own hard-won tools with them. The beauty of the human soul is a total mystery. Such an honor to have been an analyst.

Put the Christmas lights on the balcony. Like them reflected in our bedroom. Arranged crèche with all the characters from Germany, Switzerland, India, Jerusalem. Looks and smells great with the fresh pine. The choir of angels is in full voice.

Richard came over with Aidan. Adorable little boy! He loved the crèche, especially the Jerusalem donkey, carried it around with him, loved it so much he broke off its ear. I asked him if he knew what happened to my toad's crystal eye. "Ate it," he said.

Paul says Marion is into the pure magic of the Baby Jesus. First year they won't be coming for Christmas, but I know they belong there, where they will build their own home. Marion needs this Christmas—alone—to have all the time and space she needs to dream and incubate her own Mother and Child. Next year she will have a sibling.

Saw Zeca. Very hard session. His office was prepared for Christmas—soft music, fresh water, punch. I told him the last part of the saga. He was very concerned. "We'll knock it out," he said. "Don't worry. We'll knock it out and go for a completely different metabolism." We did the tests, but he said the radiation had made his results unreliable. "Persevere," Zeca said. "Think of the light in the darkness. You talk a lot about that. Now you are in it. Meditate on that." Warm with his gentle assertion, I left. Slept all the way home on the bus.

December 1, 1994

Received a very kind letter from Dr. Thomas today in response to my suggestion to Dr. Cohen that a change needs to be made at the clinic. He understands I need to change doctors. He is full of concern and hopes for my future, giving me the freedom to do what I want to do. He hopes that I "will be able to merge conventional and holistic medicine in an appropriate and effective manner." He wishes me all the best.

I thought a great deal about our relationship—relationship, yes. I have met few people who dared to be so honest with me. This is my response:

Dear Dr. Thomas,

Thank you for your letter. Thank you for your interest in me and your concern. Whatever else has happened, I have enjoyed our straightforward banter. You have from the beginning made your position absolutely clear to me. I know you are a highly respected radiation oncologist at the hospital and I have trusted and valued that knowledge.

From the beginning, you told me that you did not understand soul, relationship, love as part of the healing process. I accepted that because you put up with my pushing you, and I always felt a twinkle someplace. Now, I feel I can no longer work with you. My life is at stake. When you look at me I feel my forehead branded with DEAD across it and I feel I am dying. I know I will die if my doctor believes that I will. My body responds to your every thought. I know you don't understand that and I don't either. I do know it is a fact. Like osmosis, my cells take in what is unconsciously coming at them. Years of analytic training have helped me to shield myself, but I've never succeeded in building the shield strong enough.

So I shall seek another doctor. I do, however, thank you. I hold no resentment, no anger. I am strong and alive.

Best wishes to you,
—Marion Woodman

December 2–5, 1994

No Christmas cards this year. Trying to honor the voice that cries out within me, "Simplify. Get rid of all the conflict in your life. Get rid of 'I want to endorse my friend's manuscript. I'm too tired to read it.' 'I want to go to the conference.' 'I want to answer all those letters.'" I know there is too much breaking down of my energy that so desperately needs unity—all-out wholeness for my healing. I didn't have the cards printed in October; now I don't have the energy to address them. But how it does undo me not to connect with my friends at Christmas! Ever since I was able to write, I sat at the table with my mother and wrote Christmas cards and went to the little post office to pick them up as they came in. Well, many people are letting cards go this year. I think many are getting the message: "Simplify."

Talked to Marion. We are simplifying our Christmas as well. She says none of the children have extra money, so everyone will bring a song, a dance, whatever is creative. We'll share those and our Christmas dinner. Great! I've always hated the abundance of presents that no one can really afford and the exhaustion that undermines the meaning of the day. Soul sharing is perfect.

December 6, 1994

Another closure ritual today. Very moving—all done with different fruits. As we ate them, Lee told me what she had incorporated from her analysis. Powerful ritual. I felt great love for what we had accomplished together, then a letting go. Her purity and sincerity made me weep. "Don't worry about my tears," I said. "Better rolling down my cheeks than blocked in my kidneys."

December 8, 1994

Conference call about possibility of writing a book with Robert. I don't know how I'll ignite the fire necessary to finish a book. It's one thing puttering along with a book I'm enjoying writing; quite another seeing a deadline ahead knowing energy must be mustered to meet it—white-heat energy at that. I'm not sure that's where my energy will go, and I can no longer force it against its natural flow. Robert and Ross of course are both concerned about my health. That comes first in this valley of the shadow.

Thinking of Keats, dear John Keats, struggling to write "Hyperion" with Death in the wings:

> Or liker still to one who should take leave
> Of pale immortal death, and with a pang
> As hot as death is chill, with fierce convulse
> Die into life.

I hope I can "with fierce convulse/Die into life." The most fearful thought that whiffs through my head is of the suffering before release from cancer. I watched Mary and Sonja sweat blood with pain and Fraser's blue eyes twice their normal size. The agony became torture, ceased to have purpose. Yes, the morphine bottle was there, but so was the consciousness that demanded the dignity of their own pain. Marion, you are not yet moving toward the chill of death. Move the life imagery/energy into your cells. Convulse out of that pale, immortal world. Let the last remnants of your yearning for God-like perfection go. Cherish your imperfect humanity. Die into life.

December 9, 1994

Bizarre traffic jam on the 401 this morning, but Ross and I started out very early and made the 11:45 appointment at Princess Margaret for MRI.

Machine somewhat rounder than the one in London, less dark, less claustrophobic. Same sounds, but muffled. The technician is kind. Tentatively, I ask if it is OK. "Fine," he says. I wonder if he means the image or the result.

December 10, 1994

Breakfast with Bruce [friend]. So full of hope for his TV series on dreams. Became very excited. Felt the old creative energy. Saw myself moving into this excitement, saw myself unable to hold it, saw myself dead when the series was aired. No feeling—simply fact. I am grateful to Bruce for trying to keep me involved in the work in Toronto. It's hard for me to remember I ever wrote, ever lectured, ever ventured with my analysands into darkness beyond darkness.

Completed three closure rituals today. Felt the shuddering integrity of all three. And the letting go.

December 11, 1994

Ross and I are walking this weekend through. We don't talk about tomorrow. We get the results of the MRI and Dr.

Fyles's second opinion. We slept on and off most of the day. Several times I woke up alarmed—my breathing was so shallow I had to put my full hand on my chest and say, "It's OK, Sweetheart. It's OK. Whichever way it goes, it's going to be OK. Let the air come in. Gently. Gently."

Watch the news—Bosnia-Herzegovina, India, murders in Toronto—and wonder why I want to stay. I think the answer is for our marriage. Our work together and alone is not complete. Circumstances are forcing us into new balances in our relationship and in ourselves. Ross's wings are clipped every time he has to deal with the coffee grinder or Cascade detergent. My weight is dropping as my body ground grows stronger. Those new balances yearn to find their maturity and full flowering.

Sunny, warm December day. Bought white tulips for Charles and walked to his home. He is in worse trouble than I. Melanoma. Incredible courage! Straight talk about life and death as soon as we went in. Noreen came home, served us an essiac cocktail. She is so practical, so knowing. She gives flowers and chocolates to the nurses "just to keep things running smoothly in Charles's hospital room." She gives and demands full cooperation. Charles has come from wheelchair to crutches to cane and now faces radiation again. Ross and Charles got into their macabre black humor. We wished each other well.

> So free we seem; so fettered fast we are!
>
> —*Robert Browning,*
> *"Andrea Del Sarto"*

December 12, 1994

A card from Virginia. You know the light shining in darkness, Virginia. Thank you for the poem.

> *I have a feeling that my boat*
> *has struck, down there in the depths,*
> *against a great thing.*
>> *And nothing*
> *happens! Nothing . . . Silence . . . Waves . . .*
>
> *—Nothing happens? Or has everything happened,*
> *and we are standing now, quietly, in the new life?*
>> (Juan Ramón Jiménez, "Oceans")

That poem translated by Robert says exactly where I am today, December 12, 1994. I feel my boat has struck a great thing deep in the depths. While I was doing other things, life happened.

Worked with Dorothy until three. Then told her I was going for the verdict. Suddenly I said, "We need to recognize this moment." I felt razors on my bones. I picked up a little round Iroquois bowl and gave it to her. "The old balance will no longer hold. In this moment I am choosing to remain in this stasis or to move with confidence into the new." We saw in each other's eyes ten years of soul journeying together, both giving all to find all. We stood naked looking at each other.

Ross, Dorothy, and I went down the elevator out onto ice. Said good-bye to Dorothy at the corner, took the streetcar to Wellesley, walked in silence over the ice to Princess Margaret. I remember a fire truck screaming by, someone knocking me off the narrow path, seeing Ross ahead in his Gore-Tex coat trudging against the wind. I remember people with flowers for Christmas parties, and lovers in restaurant windows drinking coffee. As I walked, I prayed, "Dear God, do they have any idea how noble they are? Do they know how poinsettias blaze in the heart in the sheer joy of red? Do they see greenness dancing alive off Christmas trees? Do they hear the bells? Do they taste the snow? Do they smell the candles and cider?" Ross has no idea how noble he is, striding through snowflakes in the half-dark, proceeding to what is probably doom for both of us. "Dear God, for the sheer delight of incarnation, much thanks. And for the new child born in me this winter night, I thank you."

I've still a long, long time; there are still three streets more to live. . . . There are ten thousand of them, and none of them is being executed, but I am going to be executed.

—*Dostoyevsky*, The Idiot

Five more minutes—another corner to cross, another face to see, another Christmas tree alight.

When we got to the hospital, we were early, so I said, "Let's go into the Lady of Lourdes chapel. Catholics still believe in candles to burn." In we went. I prayed, "Not my will, but Thine be done." No, I did not pray that, not from the bottom of my heart. What I did pray from the bottom was "Lord, if it be Thy will, let this cup pass from me." It's a long, long, long, long way from one prayer to the other. I put lots of money in the box for candles and lit as many as I wanted to, each one a prayer for someone I love. I lit everything on the rack and my face and hands were radiant hot. Quietly, sang *Dona Nobis Pacem* to Ross and myself, and together we went into the hospital.

I looked for the first glance of Dr. Fyles. I knew I'd know before he spoke. When he came, he said, "I'm terribly sorry. I haven't received the report yet. I've been over everything else, but I need that one more report to consolidate my opinion."

That was fine with me. Could feel he was consolidating in a positive direction. So could Ross. Besides, it was another day free of doom. Home we went through streets laughing with Christmas. Slept deeply.

December 13, 1994

6:00 A.M

Awakened clear—clear as I have not been clear since last August. Can feel my body washed through, can stand straight, unclouded. Awakened with a strong inner voice saying, "Fear not." In my dream I was one of the shepherds on the hillside, terrified by the light of the angel when Christ was born. I was also myself waking up, at first frightened by the nightmare of the day ahead, then suddenly resonating with "Fear not" permeating every cell of my body. Dear God, thank you. Now I know whatever Dr. Fyles says, I do not have cancer. Or, more accurately, it is Destiny if I do. The conflict is over.

In the midst of winter, I finally learned that there was in me an invincible summer.

—*Albert Camus*, Actuelles

5:30 P.M.

Dr. Fyles met us. I knew at once he would say I was clear. "As far as I can tell," he said, "right now the tumor is benign." That's all we needed to hear. We thanked him. Came out, looked at each other, kissed, and laughed. Walked into the chapel, said our separate prayers of thanksgiving, and came to the studio. We're celebrating with salmon—a magnificent salmon that surely swam upstream, strong against the rapids, lashing its way through white water to its spawning fields.

Feel a bit strange, like a beached salmon that doesn't know quite where it's landed. Stop thinking, Bubbles. Thank God that you can ingest this invincible spirit.

December 14, 1994

Ross and I awoke early. Were on the 401 by 7:00 A.M. Love to watch dawn break over the green fields around Guelph. Hoarfrost this morning over grass and trees—"in faery lands forlorn."

> Forlorn! the very word is like a bell
> > To toll me back from thee to my sole self!
> Adieu! the fancy cannot cheat so well
> > As she is fam'd to do, deceiving elf.
> Adieu! adieu! thy plaintive anthem fades
> > Past the near meadows, over the still stream,
> > > Up the hill-side; and now 'tis buried deep
> > > > In the next valley-glades:
> > Was it a vision, or a waking dream?
> > > Fled is that music:—Do I wake or sleep?

Dear John Keats! Like the nightingale, journeying between two worlds. Driving back to London through white magic, I truly wonder, "Do I wake or sleep?" Which is the real world? In living, am I re-awakening? Or am I going back to sleep until Death calls me once again to Life? Dear God, where am I this morning? What is reality? Who am I in what reality? I am caught. I have been forever caught in the Romantic conflict. My senses pull me to the beauty of

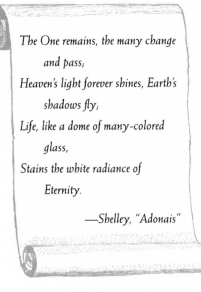

Earth; my idealism pulls me to Shelley's "white radiance." The conflict —ascendant and descendant—rages here in my sacrum.

December 15—18, 1994

Moving in No-Woman's-Land. Enjoying Christmas angels and lights. Encouraged to put up our own—the red candles in the windows—the ones we've had since we were married. They're tatty, but no others will do. Ross bought a Hallelujah Chorus poinsettia. Catherine sent a spring bouquet. The house glows. No baking this year. No open house. Many phone calls. Friends drop in. I have the only gift I need. Marion says, "All we want for Christmas is you, Auntie." And David is driving from Vancouver to be with us. They're all so sweet. We had to discourage Siobhan and Luke from coming. They were ready to spend all their money, but I'm not going to die yet.

Dear Sophia, help me to concentrate on my "holy bone." Help me to allow its heaviness to drop toward the ground, directing that energy into my feet. At the same time, help me to allow my spine to rise upward, allowing my head to float easily on top. If only people with low back pain could understand how crucial, how anguished, how magnificent that stretch can be! Our souls can magnify the Lord.

December 19, 1994

Went to see John [accountant] today. Trying to get things in order. I do my best to remember all that he says to me, but I cannot. Have to make careful notes for consideration when I come home. I hear the word "clawback" and immediately see that rampant black bear claw eight feet from my face swatting our island garbage bin across the rock. Then I realize John is silent, looking at me. I replay what my ears have heard and realize the government is the big black bear viciously about to claw back my pension. I must explain to John that the gaps are not my lack of concentration, but rather my too precise pondering on the event. I can turn that metaphorical switch off, stay with dollars and cents. But isn't it strange how people fear metaphor even though they can't speak without it?

December 20, 1994

Annual Solstice Conference Call. Talked to Saphira, Ellen, and Jean and my other Solstice Sisters. Saphira had asked us to consider: "What is the crux (cross) of the inner Sophia?" For me, now, it is the recognition of the deepest primal levels, deep connection of my pelvic bowl to the energies deep within the Earth, allowing my feet to take in that dark earth energy as love. I'm dreaming of crocodiles, turtles, flat rocks in mud, rocks that can be walked on, moved in the darkness, recognizing their light in the darkness. I'm experiencing those rocks as the wisdom in my body trying to heal itself and my dream ego as consciousness concentrating to keep my balance in the healing/devouring mud. I'm focused on the turtle's back, trying to stay on Earth, wanting to stay, not allowing my reptilian brain to carry me off to death because it cannot believe it is going to stay. My rational mind has accepted that I do not have cancer; my unconsciousness is still trapped in a death wish.

Bottom line: I am still nailed on a cross because my thinking ego is afraid to trust the wisdom of Sophia as it flows through my body into this life/death place. In almost every issue I can let go, but I am terrified of chaos. Sophia in her nether depths still feels like chaos, murderous chaos. Rather than face that killer, I fly away into rational, now archaic, patterns of thinking that need to be dumped. There's a chaos/creation out there that I want to move into.

My other crux of Sophia right now is Her connection to my new masculinity. I am moving from uterus as creative center to whole Being as creative center. The new masculine that is fighting so hard to overcome the patriarchal death sentence and the patriarchal legal stance is one half of that whole Being. His erect backbone is essential to that Being's strength; her golden bowl is essential to contain his new light. Their marriage will be consummated right there at the holy bone if I can ever find the balance.

"How would you describe the pattern that connects this to the outer world?" Saphira asks. I am at the core of my addiction. I am bringing the death wish to consciousness. Having fought so hard to live, I look at the world and a voice in me says, "Why stay in this hopeless mess?" It is Keats's exquisite nightingale and Shelley's "white radiance." The Demon Lover in his murdering perfection. He has endangered my whole life. He has also brought me to consciousness at moments of near death. As I see it, my addiction is a microcosm of the culture's addiction: The pathological idealism of Romanticism continues to murder the feminine that cherishes life. Undermined by the ensuing suicidal death wish, the culture will have to find a way to move from power drive to love, if we are to survive.

What that drive can look like in marriage is rage. "Be the ideal Mother [Father] that I want you to be or shut up. I don't want to see your chaos because it mirrors mine. So long as you pretend you're OK, I can pretend I'm OK. I'm satisfied to live the split. You be my precious Mother [Father] and I'll follow my instincts where they take me. I do not want you to live your full feminine. Your instincts embarrass me. I don't want you to live your Reality because I am too frightened to live mine. Let's stay in our safe, stifling cage of deceptive reason, drive ourselves into unconsciousness, and pretend our bodies do not exist." Is it any wonder our culture is ravaged with bodies that refuse to play host to our souls?

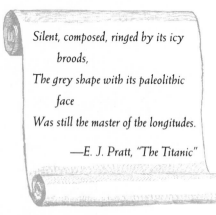

Silent, composed, ringed by its icy broods,

The grey shape with its paleolithic face

Was still the master of the longitudes.

—E. J. Pratt, "The Titanic"

My husband of thirty-six years prepared our always anniversary fillet with candles and Mozart. Cherishing sweetness of our being together for another Christmas.

December 24, 1994

Christmas Eve. Ross and I sit on the couch together after our gentle scallop supper. Decided to have our midnight mass at home, participating in the service from King's College in Cambridge (England). My body is like a piano these days: Strike a note and the full piano resonates. Those little "singer boys" with their angelic concentration and purity of tone take me right to Bethlehem.

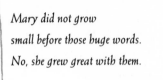

Mary did not grow
small before those huge words.
No, she grew great with them.

—Nils Peterson,
"Thinking of Mary"

Suddenly realized this is not a re-membering midnight. These hymns are searing my heart. They are all about incarnation. A virgin surren-ders to God, and when her days are accomplished, she brings forth a newborn son. In my visualizations, matter opens to receive spirit (earth energy opens to receive light vibration). A new dynamic is initiated. That dynamic eventually changes my life. God and Goddess manifesting in matter—that is incar-nation. That baby is the new consciousness: God/Goddess in every living thing—the totality of the *universe*.

This new consciousness is forcing its way into my life through illness. I am forced to experience the coming of spirit into matter and I'm just as frightened as Mary was. This newborn child turns the world into chaos. I can intuit how my life will be turned inside out after this initiation. The old questions won't matter; the old answers will be ob-solete.

This is a further answer to Saphira's question "What is the pattern that connects my present inner experience to the outer world?" The Christmas story that I have loved all my life has been incarnating itself into consciousness through illness. (No wonder I am so enraged by sentimen-tality that chooses to place Barbie dolls in the manger.)

Many of my friends and analysands are experiencing a similar transformation. They develop breakdowns of their auto-immune systems, and then slowly, slowly, slowly, in-stead of taking their body for granted, they have to bring certain areas of their body temple to consciousness. If con-sciousness flies too far ahead of matter, spirit is usually patient, slows down, allows matter to come into balance. But if matter drags its feet, symptom manifests as body turning against itself.

On the largest scale, I suspect it has to do with the chaos on our Earth. New consciousness is demanding new eyes, new ears, new antennae, new vibrations, new everything. We are microcosms of the macrocosm.

I must say, I feel like Eliot's Magi tonight! A death is in process certainly. The old dispensation no longer trusts the Holy Spirit or the Virgin Mary, or any of the images that created the Christian culture. So the new Baby sleeps on sentimental straw.

December 25, 1994

Drove back to Toronto yesterday to spend Christmas with the children. Dear Marion did her best to make a perfect Christmas. She and Richard preprepared special vegetarian dishes so there would be no hassle to get everything on the table hot. No panic at the end. They even cooked turkey pieces cut with sweet potatoes. Aidan fell this morning and punctured his tongue, so was in a bad mood. For Shelley and Guy, Christmas wasn't Christmas without roast turkey. David and Catherine were withdrawn. Quintin, Bruce, and all the Boas came on the phone from England as we were about to put everything on the table. Nothing worked according to plan. However, we celebrated. Had excellent singing with three guitars after dinner. Marion put her head on my lap as she has done on Christmas night since she was a year old. Ross and I sang carols driving through decorated Toronto as we returned to the studio.

December 26, 1994

Up early. Not a thing on the city streets or the country roads. No snow. Sunshine. Strange, eerie almost. Nothing but us and nature. Stopped at McDonald's for McMuffin and coffee. Reached Sydenham, turned on the CD, had a sparkling Boxing Day. Walked to feed the geese and ducks on the river. Lots of people in the park on roller blades. Oh, to be twenty again!

December 28, 1994

Christmas is over, but I'm feeling very close to the Christ child in my meditations. Feel new life, new hope. I can be a wise man looking at the child in the manger. I can feel the agony of his journey, his arrival at the place of the birth—a simple stable. Was he mistaken? Has everything changed or nothing? Where I am now in relation to anything, I do not know.

December 31, 1994

Ross and I had a diet ginger ale to welcome 1995.

New Year's Day, 1995

Our yearly celebration with the just-returned-from-Santa-Lucia Hamiltons—radiant with sun, flowers and fresh air. Entered the New Year transported by the Baha'i oratorio for which Ross wrote the connective narrative using parts of the Baha'i scriptures. Moved into 1995 full of hope and thanksgiving. . . . But

Still an undercurrent that I am trying to bring to consciousness. Feel like the Wise Men, who struggled so hard and so long to get to the new consciousness in Bethlehem. How did they feel when they turned around and went home? Home to what? From my small spaceship I experience everything from a new perspective. Birth yes; Death yes. Birth has brought about a Death. Sometimes when I am trying to walk on the ice lugging home a bag of potatoes, I wonder what all the fuss was about. I could have been free. Now I have to find freedom here. This is who I am in this new reality. New sensitivities, new sensibilities, new way of walking with Sophia. New focus, even on small details: fresh green romaine, not iceberg lettuce; *no* red meat, *no* wheat, or anything to which I am allergic.

Meditation happens at any moment of day or night— any time my back cries out. I stop, focus on my pelvic bowl, feel the hot energy filling the smooth porcelain and moving into my sacrum. My burning Celtic cross always appears in flames. If possible, I lie down with the bolster under my knees, allowing the energy to go through my thighs into my heels, arches, and toes. I do reflexology, cherishing my feet with lavender cream. My ankles and legs are slimmer than they have ever been. Whenever I prepare the lower ground that way, my top is full of light. Maybe Zeca is right; maybe a new metabolic process is possible in my Scotch peasant body.

Caught between two worlds—trying to move into new imagery, still not knowing what's in the bones in my back. One thing I do know: I am no longer ashamed of having been anorexic. I yearned for lightness; I still yearn for lightness. Lightness is freedom—freedom from the heaviness of too much stuff, too many words, too heavy a pull toward inertia. I feared being buried in stone—becoming stone. I yearned for bone—the lightness of bone, the stark reality of bone, the speed of bone, the beauty of bone. As a young woman I faced Medusa too directly; she petrified me, turned me to stone. Her strength was greater than mine. But now I've been forced to understand reflection—to see her in her rage, yes, but to see her in the mirror of Sophia's shield. Writing is my reflector. I'm reflecting on letting the weight of possessions go, letting the chains of outworn attitudes and rigidities go, recognizing my new responsibilities, checking what is. Present Tense IS, *esse*, verb to be, BEING. That's the feminine, right here and now in my body, my bone, my sacrum that is trying to hold the balance between light and dark, and cherish both. These roots that travel down from my five-petaled sacrum, these roots that grow through my legs and heels and feet into the core of Earth, they are growing in dark ground that makes lightness possible. Perhaps the fierce tension "Shall I stay, shall I go?" creates the tumor right in that place where the opposites meet.

Even as I write this, the roots traveling down from my five-petaled sacrum twist into twine cords. Gypsy, who was sixteen now twenty, is twisting her sweet animal body in those ropes. She grits her teeth, writhes, determined to break free. Negative Mother splays her with a look; Demon Lover strokes her forehead. Life, she wants life, nourishment, erotic union with the whole of life. Out of this black cage into freedom, freedom to BE who she IS.

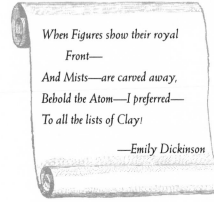

When Figures show their royal
Front—
And Mists—are carved away,
Behold the Atom—I preferred—
To all the lists of Clay!

—Emily Dickinson

I feel the lightness begin to play. Dear Emily, this is where you and I come together. "I live in possibility" was your credo. Nothing was locked in stone. Your mind delighted in images evaporating into new images. Tiny things—hummingbirds, atoms, crumbs—all carried the mystery of the universe for you. All were expressed in tiny, monumental poems. You preferred the living Atom to all the lists of Clay. And so do I.

January 2, 1995

Cold, cold day, but Mary and I did our walk out to Jack and Olga's trees in the park, and back. These Tuesday walks have become part of my earthly sustenance. I am so thankful to be able to walk that far and back. I walk naturally, gracefully, even with a certain sense of triumph.

Mary and I talked about Ruby, the lowest of the low, the scullery maid in *Upstairs, Downstairs*. In that great TV series, the hierarchy of aristocrats and equal hierarchy of their servants, Ruby, with all her fantasies of the man who would surely come to rescue her, was the scullery maid. Dear Ruby, how I loved her. Well, Ruby has reemerged in my life. Ross and I agreed that I would do the cooking and he would wash the dishes at night. After sixty years of cooking and washing up, I am weary of it. So Ross faithfully washes the dishes, but leaves the pots and pans to soak and counters covered with crumbs and spills. I ask him if he thinks Ruby will be in to finish the scrubbing. He laughs, but it makes no difference—the pans are still there. Every morning I say "Ruby wasn't on duty last night." That poor creature who takes what is dumped on her does not live here anymore. Any signs I see of her, I speak up. She is a death-trap for me.

Deathtrap because she colludes with her own victimization. Rather than confront, even quarrel, she falls into old patriarchal assumptions that are as unconscious in the man as in the woman. Seventeenth-century John Milton said it well, "He for God only, she for God in him."

But what does that look like in daily life? Who does the pots? Who cleans the bathtub? Who picks up the dirty underwear? Who is beneath the below? RUBY. Unconscious service is expected and unconscious service is given. What is the message to the feminine? Ruby will do it and Ruby is the scullery maid who scrubs in the scullery. Instead of being the heart of the home, the place of the hearth, fire, food, and transformation, the kitchen is not honored. Impossible! Ruby doesn't live here anymore.

January 3, 1995

Bruce arrived. Within a day he introduced us to things we need that we didn't know we need—thermal underwear, Hot Chili socks and mitts, new running shoes, new elements in the stove. And best of all, a present for our souls—a bird feeder on a flagpole four feet from my kitchen window. I had accepted not having my birds because we couldn't figure out how to hang a bird feeder from the second floor. Undaunted, Bruce finally got it up and the cardinals, jays, juncos, and doves were feeding almost at once. Our winter garden. Blossoms in the snow!

January 15, 1995

In a momentary leap of faith, I had my teeth fixed—fillings, cosmetic work, and a new crown. This is my body saying, "Yes, I'm going to live, so let's make me as beautiful as possible."

January 23, 1995

CAT scan. Met with Dr. James. What a new wind he is! Powerful, young king—and he knows it. Where he walks, people jump. He's trying to help me deal with this tumor in my sacrum. Such a big friendly bear!

Meditative walk at dusk. Just the snowflakes and wind and Marion coming Home. Home to Earth.

January 31, 1995

Closing ritual with Susan after four days of intense focus. She had done her homework before she came. She had gone back through her journals to the beginning of our work, picked out the primary symbols and followed them through their transformations during eight years of analysis. Each day we both felt lighter. She said she had come here expecting to be overwhelmed with grief when she left. But no. After our ritual, we were sad, but both knew the timing was right. *Kairos*, God's time, not clock and calendar. Both of us were released from personal grief through dedication to a Higher Good. Released from the past into the future. These closures take total concentration, but I am never tired afterward because Reality shimmers in the room. Realize again and again the privilege of being a midwife on these sacred journeys.

February 7, 1995

Just a little reminder of my mortality! Went to Dr. Davidson's office for my new crown. Splendid, it is! Alone, I was celebrating my new mouth by doing voice exercises in

> Then comes my fit again:
> I had else been perfect,
> Whole as marble, founded as the
>   rock,
> As broad and general as the casing
>   air:
> But now I am cabin'd, cribb'd,
>   confin'd, bound in
> To saucy doubts and fears.
>
> —*Shakespeare*, Macbeth

front of the big mirror in the main waiting room—ooing and awing as loud as I pleased from my diaphragm. Went to the bathroom. BLOOD! Macbeth in all his terror roiled up in me. Decided to say nothing to anyone unless it persists. Still, my joy was cut to flat walking on the ground mighty fast.

February 9, 1995

Final session with Dr. James, wearing his crown with such ease, blustery, seemingly in love with life.

"I'm ninety-nine percent sure it isn't cancer," he said, "but there is no way of knowing for sure what the tumor is. Neither is there any way of doing anything about it. Can't operate. No radiation, no chemotherapy. If I were you, I'd live exactly as I want to live. Go out there and do what you want to do." Frightening ambivalence in that sentence. I choose to take it positively: "Live your bliss, Marion. Vision is the best medicine for your immune system."

Thinking about psychoneuroimmunology. Conscious and unconscious have to dance together. An image, a voice, a vibration can be the link. Consciously, I surrendered, accepted the reality of death, thus resolved the conflict. Now I think my conscious mind may be the last to know that I am going to live. The hopelessness that was in my unconscious is no longer present—the green snake in my dreams is connected to the life force. But I am still looking at life through a plate-glass window. Snow White's glass coffin!

Sophia's love is the glue that can bond conscious and unconscious. I will have to faithfully wait.

Valentine's Day, 1995

Breakfast with Bruce [friend]. Worked with great excitement on his dream project for television.

Dinner with Jim. His discussion of Jung and Bohm re-
opened my knowledge of Sheldrake, Berry, and Swimme.
Different disciplines converging through archetypal fields.
That is the future!

Eating feels like learning to eat again. Music goes
through my body as if I were a piano with every string vibrating and reechoing the vibration. I can scarcely endure
the exquisiteness of a perfect note—even on a machine.
Live music is still intolerable; the edge between life and
death is right there.

When I returned to the studio tonight, I spent an hour
talking with my frightened feet. "We are afraid of being too
slow to get out of other people's way," they say. "We are
afraid of pain. We know we can't walk straight; our legs are
swinging us in." I reassure them: "Now, there is nothing to
fear. We will imagine walking straight. We have to get hold
of this immediately or we will end up toeing in like Alec
Guinness in *Richard III*, lurching around with a humped
back. Terrific technique, but not for us." Gave them a sage
bath and lavender reflexology.

February 18, 1995

Flew to Seattle. Dipping my toes in conference waters
just to see what is now right. Didn't feel like me getting in

the taxi at the front door and taking off to the airport, or taking off into the air. Didn't feel the great exhilaration— the wild sense of freedom leaving the weight of Toronto behind, flying off to a new adventure. No, nothing of that. Just plain nervous about walking at all, jealous of people who take their knee joints for granted.

"Dear Sophia, strengthen my legs, my heart, my resolve. I know your request that I speak without notes, but I would prefer to write out my speech, just this once."

"Trust," she chuckled.

Spacious room in the Mayflower Park Hotel. Trying to be here. Trying to stay in touch with Gypsy. I've lost Little One.

Hear Dr. Thomas saying, "It is quite natural for cancer patients to go into denial when metastases show up."

Hear myself fighting back, saying, "I do not believe my body is dying of cancer."

I look in the mirror for reassurance. My eyes are brighter. My posture is stronger. But then I remember saying to Dr. Fellows, "I feel so well. I don't believe it is cancer." The ropes twist on Gypsy.

Dinner with Jean. She has been a part of the prayer net that prays for me each week. So warmed by her love. Knew I was too excited to digest food, so gave up and concentrated on talking to cover up my noneating. Tomorrow rest, think about my speech, more rest.

February 20, 1995

6:00 A.M.

Long breakfast, cuddling in my corner of the dining room, watching the sleepy waiters pouring orange juice and coffee for nervous businessmen. Begin writing down notes for speech tonight. Enjoy my muffin and yogurt. Couples begin to arrive. Somehow, with strangers all around and things banging and music playing, I can rivet in on how to shape my material in a practical way. Alone in my room, I tend to become heady, theoretical. Once I have the right tone, then I need my own room to concentrate. Spent the day in silence, walked in spacious Seattle, washed my hair, did reflexology on my feet, pressed my white suit in bathroom steam, meditated with imagery.

When the soul wishes to experience something, she throws an image of the experience out before her, and enters into her own image.

—*Meister Eckhart*

Dear Sophia, as I move back into the world, help me to be fully responsible for this new sensibility. Help me to open or shield sensibly.

February 21, 1995

At 6:00 o'clock, went into gear to speak at 7:30. Picked up by a charming singer, went into the church, and from a top balcony looked down on a jammed-full auditorium. I staggered. "These people are here to hear you, Marion," I said to myself. "Yes, well, I've done my preparation. I look my best. The rest is in your hands, Sophia. Help me to be true to you and, in being true to you, true to myself. Make me an instrument of your will."

When I stood up to speak, the whole audience rose to its feet. The applause was long and

When possessed by fear, say to yourself, "I am a woman greatly loved, and capable of great loving."

—*An Ancient Crone*

deep and full of tears. I looked at them smiling and crying and clapping. I felt Sophia there before me; we were all standing in love. I had to quickly adjust inside. "Breathe, Marion, breathe into your belly. Let go. Let go. This is not a dream. It is not a memory. Breathe. These people are standing in Love." When I spoke, my voice came from a deep, quiet, natural place. Like a morning glory opening into the sun, I gradually found my full voice and full Presence and with them my sense of fun. I am strong. I am alive. Thank you, Sophia.

February 25, 1995

Came directly home. Ross met me at the airport, Precious Soul. He was listening to Ella Fitzgerald singing "Miss Otis Regrets." Two notes and I was buzzing in the bone. An older Ella—distilled, especially in her lower range. Sheer delight as she plays with the melody, gently fierce at first, then fiercely subtle as she returns to "Miss Otis Regrets." A woman who found her own voice! The trip was too much. Digestion is off, unable to walk. Need sleep, hot bath, more sleep.

But once the realization is accepted that even between the closest human beings infinite distances continue to exist, a wonderful living side by side can grow up, if they succeed in loving the distance between them which makes it possible for each to see the other whole and against a wide sky!

—*Rainer Maria Rilke*

February 28, 1995

Mostly resting, but legs are not improving. Anyway, too much ice outside to walk. Waiting to feel my own blood in my own veins, my own feet on a floor, my own fingers curling to pick up a cup—even a sense of sliding assurance that I'm not going to see my dinner plate off my lap and my food all over Mary's good carpet. Yes, waiting for the conscious knowing that I do desire turkey Tetrazzini, I do desire cranberry with lemon sauce! Even I do desire. My hands did not reach out for anything tonight.

Farewell party at Mary's for Jerry and Joan. Real loss for Ross. Jerry is such fun. Will never forget his musical gift to Ross on his 70th birthday. His rendition of Beckett and farts had everyone laughing in tears. Jerry's timing in both acting and music is exquisite. Just when he has set the stage with sentimentality and we're all weepy waiting for the sweet note, he hits a "wrong" one. No hassle! Carry on. *C'est la vie.* A brilliant clown holds the comedy at the core of the tragedy.

Detachment is the move from tragedy to divine comedy—seeing the as-it-is, even the nobility in the suffering of humanity. When I was midwife for Sonja in her dying, she said to me, "Pull out those tubes, Marion. Give me the dignity of my pain." No more IV, no more morphine. I *witnessed* her anguish. Together we honored her pain and through our honoring, everything nonessential to soul was stripped away. "How two souls can love each other," she said. Every inch a queen!

March 5, 1995

Snowdrops—five tufts of sweetness in our garden! Dear Sophia, tell me why I cannot dance, why I cannot walk. I know I do not have cancer, but something is very wrong.

Sophia:	Marion, you know there are lessons to be learned. You love dancing. You think of yourself—light, fast, free—free of earth, free of bondage to your body. In your "perfect" body, you are in control, addicted to the light that keeps you out of body. You're a swan maiden, addicted to wings, addicted to spirit. You refused to eat in order to fly.
Marion:	But I moved into my body almost thirty years ago when I was faced with Death in India. When Death stared me in the eye, I wanted to stay here on Earth.
Sophia:	True. But we're moving into another level of the spiral. The lack of balance between Earth and Heaven is what's causing the tumor in your sacrum. Your edema now is mirroring the rise of your unconscious as it did twenty-five years ago. That is your Achilles' heel. You have to understand in your bones that life in your father's garden at the age of three belongs to the age of lower innocence. The age of perfection! Edema kept you heavy even when you couldn't eat either food or images and forced you, literally and figuratively, out of your Father's house. Like Noah, you built an ark to save you from the flood. That ark was consciousness—your covenant with God. But you still believed that *I am that I am* was in control and you who worshiped Him were also in control. There's a new lesson in control. Go and read "The Clod and the Pebble."
Marion:	I see what you mean. I don't like being "a little Clod of Clay,/Trodden with the cattle's feet." Interesting, one of my repetitive experiences as a child, even into adulthood, was of three Here-

ford cows who accompanied me wherever I went. They were my unconscious Good Mother who protected me. They were always there with great placid eyes, chewing, always chewing, watching—ever watching. The cattle in the streets of India brought the Herefords into consciousness. Just realized I never dreamed of them again. Their protection was transformed into the cherishing of the dark Indian woman whose warm arm held me in life in the Ashoka Hotel. The dark woman became the Black Madonna of my dreams, and thence to You. Thank you for guiding me through my stumbling. Help me to be strong enough to surrender certainty. To leap into the mystery. Help me build "a Heaven in Hell's despair."

The Clod & the Pebble
"Love seeketh not Itself to please,
Nor for itself hath any care;
But for another gives its ease,
And builds a Heaven in Hell's
despair."

So sang a little Clod of Clay,
Trodden with the cattle's feet;
But a Pebble of the brook,
Warbled out these metres meet:

"Love seeketh only Self to please,
To bind another to its delight;
Joys in another's loss of ease,
And builds a Hell in Heaven's de-
spite."

—William Blake

If only I could release Gypsy from her bindings, pull her into consciousness, let the terror of annihilation go! At the same time, Swan Maiden has to sacrifice her wings. Gypsy comes up from darkness to meet Swan coming down from Light. If they could come together, I might be whole. Surrender, Marion. Be a lily of the field, even a little clod.

March 6, 1995

Talked to Martin today and to Bob [two doctor friends]. Maybe I'm projecting, but I think they both think I am in denial. When I say, "I feel steady," they say, "That's good. Keep trying." I am aware of my capacity for denial, but I think I am better. Still, I must acknowledge something is strange in my behavior. I am incapable of obeying a clock, I who was once so punctual. I am not confused though I may appear to be. I tell people I will meet them at a certain time, but then I cannot hurry. I know I am going to be late, but something in me does not care. I am doing my best and can do no more. I may not get there at all. I feel no guilt, no remorse. I'm on different time.

> What is not brought to consciousness comes to us as Fate.
>
> —C. G. Jung

March 8, 1995

Edema is heavy again. When my body fills with water, I dream of troops manning all the posts against the enemy who is pounding at a plate-glass door. Plate glass is cut-off from feeling—able to watch life, unable to feel into it. Whatever strength is in me takes up water (unconsciousness) to protect against the enemy (life itself). Good image for autoimmune breakdown: Body becomes enemy to itself. Sooner or later, I hope that plate glass will shatter: Swan

Maiden will sacrifice her impossible ideals and accept Gypsy with her luscious love of life. One comes out of Light to meet the Other coming out of Darkness. Sometimes I hear Little One laughing when I write a sentence like that. I suspect she is a very old crone.

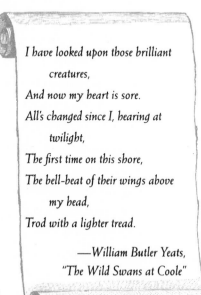

> And the Word was made flesh, and dwelt among us.
>
> —*John I*

March 15, 1995

Martin phoned this morning: "I hear the wild swans in the sky as they make their way to Grand Bend." Ross and I have never seen them, so we drive up about 4:00 P.M. wondering if we will see anything. As we come close to the water, we can hear a few calls—higher-pitched than Canada Geese, more like laughter than cackling. Then we begin to see a few lines of birds flying in formation. A few, but disappointing. Then we drive to a farm, near a lagoon. The road runs right beside it. We drive up to the back field and get out of the car. Hundreds—in fact, we're told fifteen thousand were there last night—resting and feeding on their way north. What glory! As they rise from the cornfield to fly to the water, they are right over our heads, maybe fifteen feet above us. We can see the lace of their wings, pristine white, and hear their sad call, sad and sometimes funny at the same time.

> *I have looked upon those brilliant*
> *creatures,*
> *And now my heart is sore.*
> *All's changed since I, hearing at*
> *twilight,*
> *The first time on this shore,*
> *The bell-beat of their wings above*
> *my head,*
> *Trod with a lighter tread.*
>
> —*William Butler Yeats,*
> *"The Wild Swans at Coole"*

Such elegance—every one in perfect formation position, flying full stretched. As we look toward the west, the sky is dark blue, the rose pink of the sunset tinged with living gold and the golden rays of the setting sun connecting to the water. As the lines of swans fly into the sunset, they are white crests on elongated ocean waves, their wings moving in slow rhythm like the everlasting motion of the waters. Unforgettable, mystical, they

> *Begin, and cease, and then again begin,*
> *With tremulous cadence slow, and bring*
> *The eternal note of sadness in.*
>
> (*Matthew Arnold, "Dover Beach"*)

March 16—17, 1995

Went alone to the university symposium on cancer and diet. Didn't learn much. Repeat, repeat on green and yellow vegetables. Green tea is good, also wheatgrass and vegetables of the sea. Do not eat barbecued food because the charred part is very bad, as is the charred part in frying and searing. All damned white sugar, white flour, refined foods in general. Eliminate fat and sugar as much as possible, except for olive oil and canola oil.

All emphasized the importance of diet. Irony! What I'll remember most about the conference was the fabulous coffee and muffins.

Gypsy is alive and well! "The eternal note" resonates from yesterday. All is as-it-is. And that's OK.

Simplifying becomes my total focus. I'm noting how anxious I become when I fail to simplify or cannot simplify because of what starts happening around me—phone, TV, letters, ad infinitum. I believe that failure to simplify could lead me back into cancer because I would lose touch with my life vibration—my tone that sustains my life force. In my hours with analysands, one of my strong points has been my capacity to filter irrelevancies, to listen for their essence. Yes, we blow out anger, jealousy, fear, knowing that negative energy brought to consciousness can transform into creative energy. However, searching for garbage in the psyche is no longer relevant when soul is living its essence—being seen, being heard. Anxiety is stripped away by concentrated listening and perceiving. Concentrated vision operating in all the senses is what I mean by simplifying.

The more I listen to my soul, the more clearly I hear the truth of other people, of animals, birds, the universe. A unified field! One clear melody—like the song of a cardinal—sings out, and everything else fades away. The simplifying happens. Real issues become clear. This is why Mozart's music is so important to me now. Like a clarion, a melody comes to me in its full spectrum and opens my full spectrum. The unimportant falls away. Healing happens. The music reestablishes the healthy frequency.

I must stay in touch with whatever keeps me focused on the still point—the place of exact harmony in body and psyche. Simplify life to that point where the dance can happen—the dance between consciousness and the unconscious. So long as I constantly allow other things to interfere, I will never find the moments in each day to reach those listening points of harmony—those seeing points of perception. Concentration that can focus on the moments must come first or the others do not follow. I tend to think I'll get everything in order and then. No, no, no! That's not it. Listen to Mozart first, come into harmony first, then clutter will fall away unnoticed.

Clarification is very important now because I know the dance is not happening. The swans have flown into the sunset; Gypsy is alive. But consciousness and the unconscious are not dancing together. The unconscious is ready to step into life; consciousness *knows* I can move into health, but dares not leap into the unknown. I cannot walk.

March 31, 1995

Paul phoned at 6:30 A.M. to tell us that Emma Sophia was born yesterday at 8:23 P.M. on the cabin floor. With him were Marion Rose, Susan, and two midwives. Everything went smoothly. Kathryn came on the phone, delighted to have borne her second child in natural childbirth. She described Marion being so interested, so intense, a part of everything. In the most critical moments she tore off her clothes and threw herself naked over her mother's breast saying, "Push, Mamma, push."

Everything in me rejoiced for her. Imagine how different my life would have been, and Father's and Mother's, and my brothers', if instead of surgery and aloneness, we had been a part of our mother's body as she gave birth. If only she had been able to rejoice, and Father and I, instead of each of us separately enduring whatever we endured alone. To see the feminine vagina open and present the miracle of a baby—to experience life as miracle! I feel Marion's awe. What a gift on the cabin floor!

I think of the innocence of that little child coming into the end of this millennium, as this civilization is breaking up. I wonder what she will see in her lifetime. All my love goes out to her. I look at my black sapphire with the light radiating within and I pray to God that she will be able to see that light. She carries the name of the Goddess who will be brought to consciousness in the new millennium. She may be called Acausal, Nonlocal, Synchronicity, Chaos—the name doesn't matter.

The plate glass that was around me is now a rainbow. The rainbow is dancing molecules of red, green, yellow, lilac, and lily of the valley. Color and form, sight and smell, even textures and tastes are juxtaposed.

I always associate rainbows with subtle body: rainbow as connection between Earth and Heaven; subtle body as connection between matter and spirit. Constant shifting in my dreams; the images are too new to grasp.

To Herman and Kirtley's for dinner with their three children. Memories of family sitting down to turkey dinner. I began to mention the many dinners I had cooked. Herman burst into laughter. "Marion, you don't cook." And he believed it. He never associated me with a kitchen, cooking, cleaning. Few people do. We rarely entertain now. But time was when I served dinner (everything homemade) to forty to fifty people. The theater closing night parties, the glorious Christmas parties with all the children in the pageant, the elegant dinners after I took the course in Old London at the Cordon Bleu. Ah, yesterday!

April 1, 1995

Between the form of Life and Life
The difference is as big
As Liquor at the Lip between
And Liquor in the Jug

The latter—excellent to keep—
But for ecstatic need
The corkless is superior—
I know for I have tried

(Emily Dickinson)

Went to Henrikus's 50th birthday party. Too difficult to walk from car to house. Living room full of laughing faces, platters laden with fine *cheeses*, breads, sweets. And tulips, tulips, tulips as only the Dutch can grow. We talk quietly to everyone. Don't move from the safety of the couch. Very tired. At 10:30, we are about to leave.

As we reach the very threshold of the front door (five minutes earlier and the story would have been very different), to my surprise and delight, a sixtyish Dutchman with Dutch sailor cap strides through the open door playing a tuba. Then another of the same ilk, and another, and another—twelve, all playing trumpets and trombones, or some other brass, all dressed in "Tomato Soup" long coats with bright yellow lapels and cuffs. The room rocks with polkas, waltzes, fox-trots. I haven't dared to dance for three years. Ross and I return to the couch. I can barely endure listening.

"Come on, Ross," I finally say. "Let's dance."

"Oh, Marion," he says, "you know you can't dance. You could break your back."

I sit out the polka, can't keep my feet still. They remember—oh how they remember tapping it out in South Porcupine, Timmins, Schumacher, Heidelberg, Rüdesheim, Grinzing, yes, even Old London. I feel like Death sitting there with all my life past. Then my hands are clapping like a child's. The energy builds, becomes so fierce I feel like a puppet with hands and feet tapping syncopated rhythms, feet doubling in toe and heel. Puppet becomes young woman, vibrant with animal energy. A voice comes up from my perineum, "Marion, you can sit on this couch until you rot, but I am going to dance. I don't care what Ross thinks. I don't care what these Dutch-Canadians think. I don't care what anybody thinks. I don't care if you break your back. I don't care if you drop down dead. I am going to dance! I am going to live!" I feel the archetypal energy lifting me off the couch, propelling me across the room—I feel it pushing through my benumbed feet, legs, thighs, torso, arms, hands, through every cell into my head. It is TOTAL. I feel myself Gypsy—a twenty-four-year-old glowing woman. I am being danced. People are gazing at me aghast, probably thinking, "This old lady sat on the couch all evening; suddenly she's transformed into a hands-in-the-air gypsy. What's she up to?" Do I care?

I become concentration. Then a stranger—a Dutchman who has just arrived—catches my vision, jumps into my circle, and we dance a dance as fierce as I have never danced before. If my back breaks, if I drop dead, it doesn't matter. I am twenty-four. I am healthy. I am whole.

Happy 50th, Henrikus. I'll never forget this birthday.

Thank you, dear Sophia. From every cell in my broken body, my radiant body, I thank you. I am alive. I am free . . . to live . . . to die.

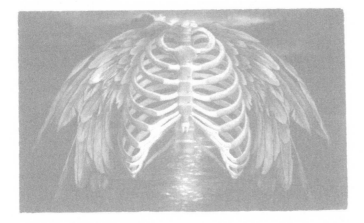

AFTERWORD

I had never read Marion's journal, not that I was forbidden, but that I knew my mind did not belong there. Marion also knew it. Before I woke up in the morning, she would already be in her room writing. Not yet awake, I would reach over and find her gone. That's how my day would begin.

By breakfast time, Marion's day was in full motion. Mine had not yet begun, except as the shock of her absence. Marion was about some other business that included me without being about me. It was about Marion in herself where anyone, including me, would be an intruder. Except, of course, God, or closer still, Sophia. I only remotely understood how close that closeness was. It was some distance from myself.

Her eagerness even before coffee never ceased to surprise me. It was like an alarm clock going off, waking me from a deep sleep. My temptation was to turn it off and go on sleeping. Marion knew that talking to me first thing in the morning was largely talking to herself. The journal was between us like a sword. It was neither a severing nor a wound, but a sharpness of discretion that had to be removed before we could join. Both Marion and I, each in our different way, respected the mystery of the other. We negotiated with that into a relationship that was profound.

Finally one morning Marion came with her journal. She said she wanted to read some of it out loud. I was startled into a more fully awakened state. She read to me about her cancer. And I knew why. She had felt my withdrawal and she knew if I didn't soon get here, here to where she was, I might lose her without quite knowing, until too late, what was happening, or had already happened. Marion was letting me into a place I had never been. She was stepping into an absence that was, oddly, an absence in myself where I had thought I did not belong. It was a place of trauma, the fear that she might be gone forever.

The soul's journey with Marion, our journey together, together and apart, had been painful and insightful beyond my expectation. At times I wanted out. But out of what? I was in deep enough to know: out of my own feminine soul, always a stranger to me. Always, in a sense, an absence that I needed, not necessarily wanted, to fill. Marion was that, increasingly that, to me. There was no out to get out of except out of myself. Cancer brought this spiritual matter to a head, though I seemed unable to face it. The fear of death was not only Marion's death. It was my own, my own soul death. While Marion wrote in her journal I had slept, awakening to an absence that seemed well beyond my reach.

Our relationship had for both of us always demanded change, which Marion thought of as surrender as distinct from compromise. Surrender was Marion's word, her word for the feminine soul that she thought of as a Pregnant Virgin, the soul pregnant with its own virgin life. I thought it belonged to her, to the Marion of her journal, not to me. I was not quite sure what belonged to me.

Cancer brought all this to a head. What all along I had been in search of, though mainly as one asleep, was in Marion's cancer journal, parts of which she decided, now or never, one morning to read to me. The time had come for a meeting in a place we had never really met, for me a place of absence that I nevertheless needed to fill. It was somewhere well beyond the rational shallows of my mind.

In the very midst of Marion's dying I had sat one evening on a couch and, terrified, I watched her dance knowing that her spine might crack. I saw at that moment only the X-rayed tumor at its base that we now assumed was benign. But my terror was also her joy. Someone else, a stranger, took her in his arms and danced with her from room to room. It seemed that he was the stranger in myself, my own fear, terror even, of soul.

Gradually, reading the journal again and yet again, the terror has departed. I now feel I know the stranger in myself. In Marion's dance of life I think I have finally joined her. Our bodies in their wondrous decrepitude sway together to a music that joins our shared beloved earth to other, no longer distant, or quite so distant, spheres.

—Ross Woodman